ENERGIZE

An Hachette UK Company
www.hachette.co.uk

First published in Great Britain in 2009 by Hamlyn,
an imprint of Octopus Publishing Group Ltd
Carmelite House
50 Victoria Embankment
London EC4Y 0DZ
www.octopusbooks.co.uk

This edition published in 2019 by Pyramid, an imprint of Octopus Publishing Group Ltd

Distributed in the US by
Hachette Book Group
1290 Avenue of the Americas
4th and 5th Floors
New York, NY 10104

Distributed in Canada by
Canadian Manda Group
664 Annette St.
Toronto, Ontario, Canada M6S 2C8

ISBN 978-0-7537-3355-4

A CIP catalogue record for this book is available from the British Library.

Printed and bound in China

10 9 8 7 6 5 4 3 2 1

For the Pyramid edition:
Publisher: Lucy Pessell
Designer: Lisa Layton
Artworker: James Pople
Editor: Sarah Vaughan
Production Controller: Grace O'Byrne

ENERGIZE

spring clean your mind and body to get
your bounce back today and every day

JO SALTER

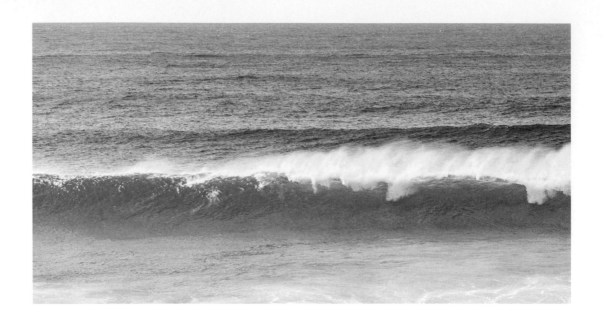

ABOUT
THE
AUTHOR

Jo Salter MBA is a renowned motivational speaker, using boundless vitality, humour, compassion and understanding to provide practical advice and inspiration to audiences internationally. Britain's first female fast-jet pilot, and a mother of two, Jo was voted by *Harpers and Queen* magazine as "one of the 50 most inspiring women in the world".

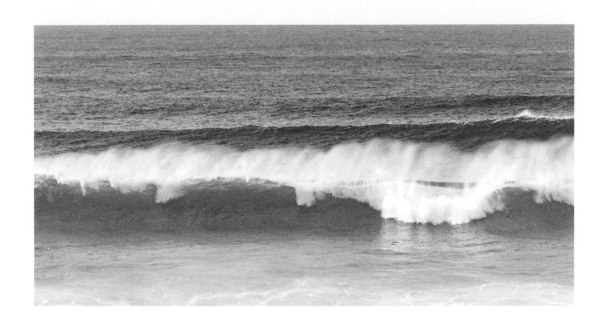

CONTENTS

Introduction   6

The energy factor   8

Energy profiles   22

Energy techniques   46

Energy, here I come!   120

Index   126

Acknowledgements   128

INTRODUCTION

Energy is vital. We all need energy, whatever our aims,
however we feel. I am delighted to share what
I know about energy and energy sources with you.

Energy has been of vital importance to me throughout my life and career. Looking back, I can see that I have thought, read and talked about energy in many different ways – meditating while lying in bed fraught with teenage angst, responding to stressful situations while flying a fast jet at a few hundred feet above the ground at 600 mph, and preparing myself to give an inspirational speech to over a thousand people. I remember the stress of those first years of parenthood, when there was little sleep to be had. Of course, different events in my life demanded differing levels of energy and skill – but I needed the energy to develop, to use and to keep up those skills.

ENERGY DEMANDS

Whoever we are, 21st-century living puts massive demands on us – whether it be balancing our work and personal lives, coping with the rising cost of living or dealing with people and environments that sap our energy. Many of us find ourselves exhausted by modern life – rushing from one part of our busy lives to the next, supplementing real energy with caffeine and other quick pick-me-ups.

ENERGY SOLUTIONS

There is a solution for anyone who needs more energy. I have written this book to help you improve the quality of your life. It will provide you with the tools to assess your current energy levels and then design your own personalized plan to deal directly with your needs. There are many types of energy. As you read this book, you will discover your six energy profiles – physical, emotional, intellectual, creative, personal and spiritual. You will also learn about your overall energy profile, which helps you to see yourself as a balanced whole, understanding the balance of your energy profiles – or, if not, to identify where the imbalance lies.

This book packages together a plethora of ideas, tips, strategies and lifestyle choices that will help you regain your energy, from the basic energy techniques that we develop as children, such as good sleeping, eating and exercising habits, to exercises that help you think more creatively and how to develop meditative techniques.

HOW TO USE THIS BOOK

It is a good idea to keep the first overall energy profile sheet you draw up as you can come back and answer the questions again in a few weeks' or months' time and compare the two. You could even draw your goals on the sheet to give you something to work toward. There are many tools to help you on your way to a more energized you. Use as many as you can.

The techniques in the book come from a variety of sources: things my grandmother used to say, tips from friends and family, information digested from reading many books, and some that I have created for my personal use from my experience as both a fast-jet pilot and a motivational speaker. The techniques are not prescriptive, but offer you a choice of methods to ensure that you can fulfil your needs in the way you want to.

Make a commitment to yourself here and now. Accept that you are accountable to yourself for your improvement. Ask friends and family to support your efforts and use the tools and techniques in this book to help you rediscover the complete energized you. It takes energy to enjoy the world and live life to the full. Taking a few steps at a time, you will find yourself energized, capable and full of joy.

Carpe diem – seize the day! Enjoy!

THE ENERGY FACTOR

This chapter provides an overview of energy itself and the impact that the different stages of life have on one's energy levels. Life is full of energy-sappers, and recognizing these "red flags" is crucial to avoiding them (see pages 20–21). You may want to make your way straight there and see whether you recognize any of them in your life; or you could do the questionnaire (see pages 26–29) in the "energy profiles" section to carry out your own energy self-assessment, and then check back on the red flags to see where your profile and energy needs meet.

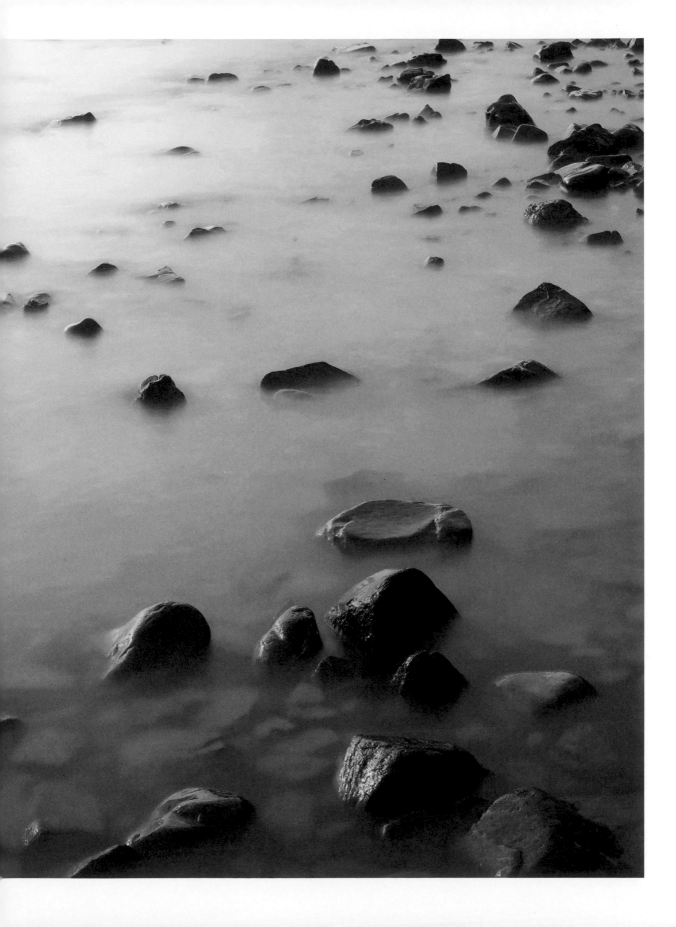

WHAT IS ENERGY?

The world is a ball of energy. Look around you. Everything you can see is made up of energy. You can see the different shapes of trees, or objects, or people. However hard you look, though, your eye cannot see the constituent parts that make up everything in our world. If you break these parts down enough, you are left with pure energy. Aside from these tangible objects, we are surrounded by invisible energy all the time in the form of radio and television waves transmitted to our homes 24 hours a day, seven days a week. There are waves of energy in sunlight and in sounds that we cannot pick up within the normal human hearing range.

ENERGY AROUND THE WORLD

Life in the 21st century is busy and there is precious little time in which to stop and recharge. Despite this, important threads are emerging from modern thinkers that highlight the importance of understanding energy and using it to our benefit. However, this is not a new phenomenon and the subject of energy has been studied around the world in many different cultures. Here is a brief outline of the different energy disciplines and ways to think about energy.

Acupuncture inserts needles into the body, often along the energy meridians, or at specific points, to treat pain and improve health.

Ayurvedic medicine is a system of traditional medicine that has been practised in India for thousands of years. It is devised from two Sanskrit words, "Ayus" meaning life and "Veda" meaning knowledge, so "Ayurveda" is the knowledge of life. It focuses on maintaining a balance of energies rather than on the symptoms themselves and applies to the mind, body and spirit as a whole.

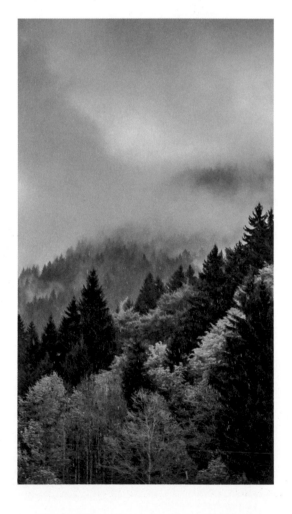

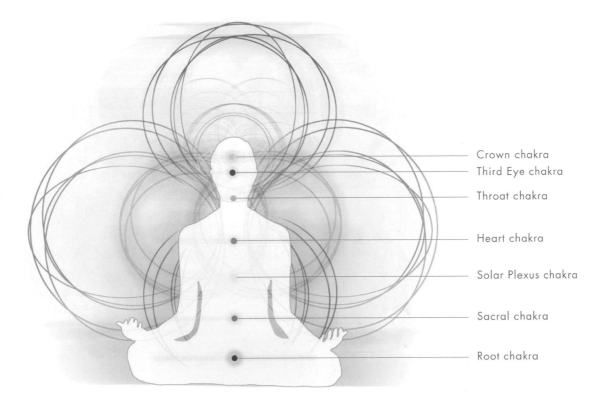

Crown chakra
Third Eye chakra
Throat chakra
Heart chakra
Solar Plexus chakra
Sacral chakra
Root chakra

Chakras Chakra is a Sanskrit word meaning "wheel", and refers to one of the seven centres of our energy system. The chakras are the Root, Sacral, Solar Plexus, Heart, Throat, Third Eye and Crown. Each have their own associated consciousness and body–mind associations.

Chi or qi, or "vital energy", has been studied by the Chinese for thousands of years. It is the concept of air or breath – the energy or vital essence of both an individual and the individual when linked to the vast energy of the universe itself. The Chinese have analysed patterns of energy within the human body and plotted 12 channels of chi. These meridians correspond with the major organs of the body, and are: lung; large intestine; stomach; spleen; heart; small intestine; urinary bladder; kidney; heart constrictor; triple heater; gall bladder; liver. If there is a break in the flow between these

meridians, then there is an imbalance in the body and an individual's energy levels will suffer. This is used for both preventative health care and for treatment of diseases, where disease is seen as a blockage in the energy channels. This meridian system of healing is used in herbal therapies, massage, acupuncture and Shiatsu (see next page).

Flow/zone A sense of being in the energy zone, or in the flow of energy, has been reported by athletes and high-performing individuals. It describes a point where an individual is absorbed in an activity, totally focused and in touch with his or her abilities in an almost effortless way. It is a point of peace and complete energy.

Indian head massage, also known as "champissage", is based on the Ayurvedic system. It relieves stress and tension and is said to affect the three higher chakras of the Throat, Third Eye and Crown.

Massage is renowned for its health benefits, in terms of treating both body and soul.

Positive thinking is a way of thinking that colours everything in a positive light. Thoughts, language and visualizations are all focused on positive, successful and happy outcomes, with the expectation of receiving what you think about. The "law of attraction" is based on a similar concept, namely that you attract whatever you think about into your life. The more you think about something, the more likely it is to arrive.

Qigong combines the chi discussed above with achievement and self-discipline. It is practised through meditation, movement and breathing exercises that integrate the mind and body, remove toxins from the body, reduce stress and, of course, improve energy levels.

Reiki is a Japanese term for universal life energy. It is a way of healing by passing energy through the hands; the energy travels to where it is needed in the body. It is a holistic healing energy for the mind, body and spirit. It is also said to fill the aura, an energy force that some people report to see as an individual's life-force.

Science Energy has been studied as a science for many years and there are some well-known energy equations and laws:

- $E = mc^2$
- potential energy = mgh
- kinetic energy = $\frac{1}{2} mv^2$
- First law of thermodynamics: energy cannot be created or destroyed, but is transformed.
- Second law of thermodynamics: every time you do work, some energy is lost as heat.
- Third law of thermodynamics – there is no such thing as a perpetual-motion machine.

Shiatsu is working on the affected meridian or pressure point until any blockages are released and the energy flow can return.

Synchronicity is a term, created by Carl Jung, that means unexplained yet meaningful coincidences.

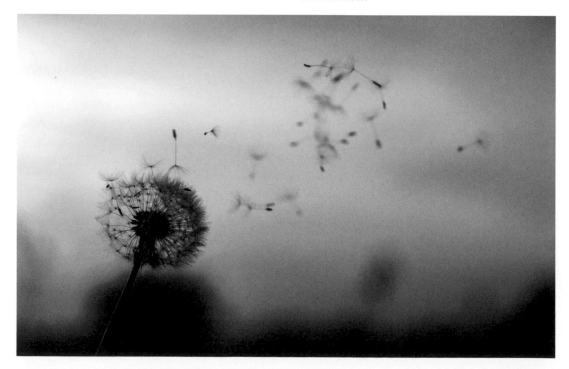

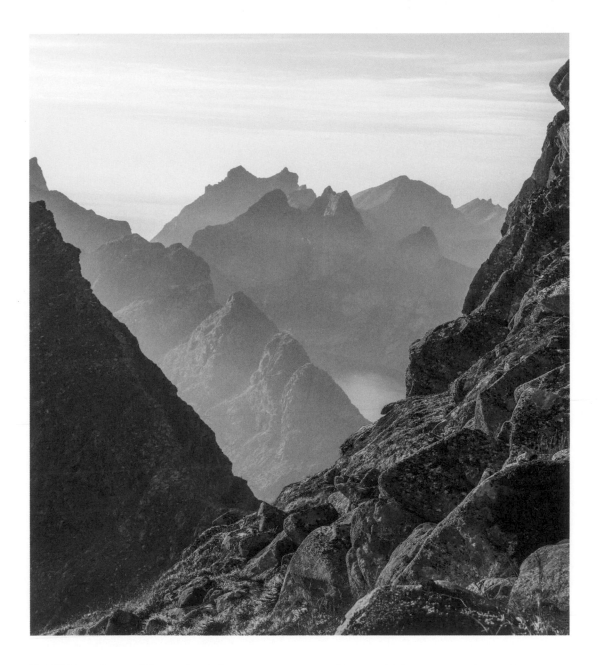

Tai Chi is an internal (internal as it focuses on mind, spirit and chi) Chinese martial art, practised for "purposes of health and longevity", and is a form of Qigong (see previous page). It is about slow movements, balance and awareness – both at a physical and mental level.

Universal energy As we are all made up of energy, we are all linked with everything else on the planet and in the universe. Therefore,

anything we think or act upon has an impact on the overall universal energy flow. The theory is that asking the universe, or "cosmic ordering", may help your dreams to become reality.

Yin yang The yin-yang symbol is well known across the world. The symbol shows the opposites of feminine and masculine, dark and light, yet they remain connected and each contain an element of the other.

UNDERSTANDING ENERGY

When someone is "full of energy", it is easy to picture an individual rushing around with high physical levels of energy or perhaps talking very quickly. While there is no doubt that this person is expending a great deal of energy, if the energy is not focused, he or she may find themselves "shedding more heat than light".

PSEUDO-ENERGY

This is unfocused energy. It is important to recognize the difference between pseudo-energy and controlled, calm energy. It comes in many forms – think of the calm of Gandhi and what he achieved. His energy was focused. Think of traders, doctors or schoolteachers who manage a class of children – they would not be able to do their jobs without controlled and focused energy that enables them to respond to the needs of the moment.

RECHARGING THE BATTERIES

Part of my job is to give inspirational talks. I was once introduced for such a talk by a man who had so much energy and enthusiasm that he appeared mildly hysterical. He gestured me on stage, clapped wildly, then shot off and left me to talk to a stunned audience. The result was a "burn-up" of energy in the room. The audience had been left drained. My only option was to re-energize the room before starting my planned talk. I started with a relaxation exercise, giving people the time to reach their own inner core and refuel. I then continued with my speech, making sure I included an overview of understanding energy and an introduction to the audience of a technique to overcome energy-draining situations.

BEHAVIOUR HABITS

Habits influence our behaviour, and behaviour is set by habits, but we frequently link the word habit with negativity – a "habitual gambler" or a "smoking habit". Habits can work for and against us, since they can also be associated with positive behaviour. Habits form unconsciously all the time. It can be difficult to consciously acquire good habits or dispose of bad ones, and doing so can require great discipline.

Why not try something now that will make you feel good and make it your first step towards conscious habit-forming? Go and do something to make you laugh, enjoy a walk in beautiful surroundings or be with people who make you feel good. Link your new habit to one you carry out every day, such as cleaning your teeth.

THE ENERGY EQUATION

In a simple form, energy can be represented as:

energy = sleep + water + nutrition + exercise + attitude

So, if you make sure you get enough sleep, drink sufficient water, eat well, exercise and think positively, you will be energized.

EXPERIENCING ENERGY

To truly understand something, you need to experience it. How we experience energy depends on our personal view of the world as well as the emotional or physical state we are in at any time. There are times when we feel irritable, although there does not seem to be a direct cause. Instead of accepting this, try to dissociate yourself so that you can judge and be aware of the different effect situations, people, food, stress, anxiety or laughter have on you and your energy levels. Self-awareness and understanding of these energy flows is a big step forwards and change can quickly follow.

To experience the simplest form of energy, go to your local beauty spot and stop and be still. So often, a feeling of peace will come over us. If you cannot get out somewhere now, remember a time when you felt peaceful and energized – try to recreate that feeling and make opportunities to relive it whenever possible.

Sometimes, we can capture energy when laughing with friends or being engrossed in a book or a piece of music. For a moment, everything feels perfect. Capture that feeling and anchor it in your mind, as this is the point you should come back to when you need to re-energize. Anchoring is a useful technique to help you evoke positive feelings and memories. Useful guidance tips on positive visualization can be found in the techniques section (see page 94).

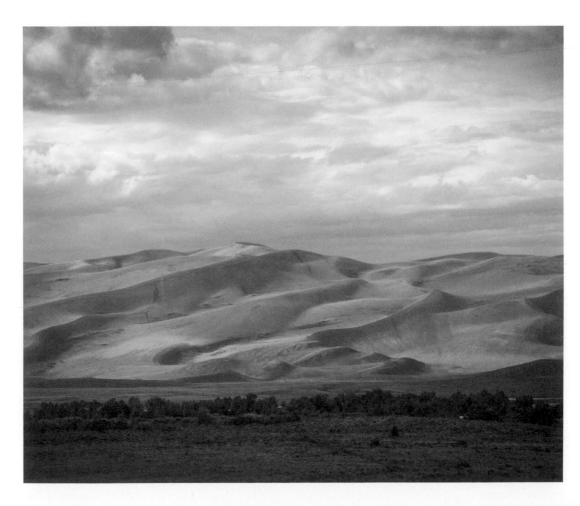

FULFIL YOUR EXPECTATIONS

Setting realistic expectations can be difficult. Whether we are setting them too high or too low, it can cause disillusionment and demotivation. Being aware of where you are and where you want to be is the first step. It may be that just one step is all you need to take. For others, only a long jump might be enough – it depends on you and what your needs are.

PRACTICE MAKES PERFECT

It is important to find the appropriate energy for the appropriate time. There is no advantage to firing yourself up when it is time to sleep, just as low energy levels are not useful when you need a focused mind for an exam.

It is better to exercise for ten minutes every day than to rush out and over-extend your body by working hard for an hour and then not be able to do any exercise for the next few months.

There is an ideal energy-level line plotted in the Appropriate Energy diagram given below that shows where you want to be at various times. Watch out for burn-out – there is only so long we can work at optimum performance.

APPROPRIATE ENERGY

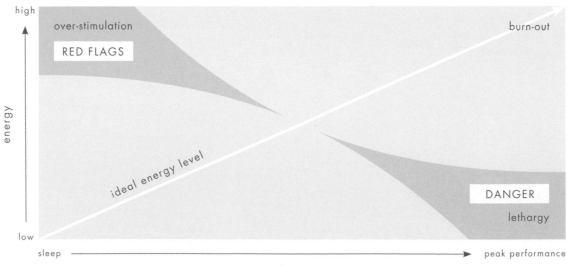

PERSONAL FULFILMENT

This book is about you. What is it that motivates you? What challenges your willpower and self-control? What could you do to help yourself and what do you want for yourself? Take some time to visualize the sort of person you want to be and then work on achieving your goals.

Personal fulfilment is often linked to achievement, so it is important for us to manage our time and pursue goals that are meaningful to us. We live in a frenetic world where we often don't have time to do simple things. We are constantly exposed to media images and bombarded with information. It can be hard to distinguish between the necessary and unnecessary. Whether your goals are ambitious (pursuing world peace) or immediate (getting to work on time), managing these goals and taking steps to achieve them will lead to satisfaction and fulfilment.

SPHERE OF INFLUENCE

A common frustration people experience is trying to instigate change and finding that nothing happens. This is often because the person concerned is trying to exert influence in an area where they have none. There is a simple technique that will help you ensure that you don't waste your energy in this way.

Imagine there is something in the workplace you would like to change. Consider your sphere of influence. Draw a circle and put your name inside. Draw another circle around that one and write down all the names of people you can influence. Finally, draw another circle around the two circles and write down names of the people you cannot influence. Now stop and think about the outcome you want. Who can you influence? What could you do about it? What would you

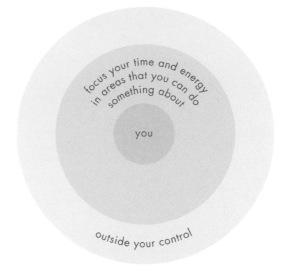

need to do to get a key individual into your sphere of influence?

If the thing that you would like to change is completely out of your control, don't waste your energies on it, but find an alternative project or a different path. Focus on what you can influence rather than on things outside your control.

FINISH WHAT YOU START

How many times have you started something and then not finished it? The sense of having lots of unfinished projects is de-energizing. Work on improving your self-discipline and willpower so that you complete tasks. Break the task down into a series of stepping points and reward yourself when you achieve them.

In the real world, you cannot do or have everything, however much you may want to. It is important to accept this and focus on what is most important to you. Balance your energies; work in moderation to achieve what is most important rather than overdo things pursuing unnecessary goals.

THE RIGHT TYPE OF ENERGY

We all need different energy levels at different times. The energy required to sit and focus on research in a library is very different from that needed to play an energetic sport. Just as we need different energies for different activities, we need different energies for the different phases of our life.

BIORHYTHMS

One idea is that our lives are based on three biological rhythms or cycles: emotional, intellectual and physical. When plotted (based on your birth date), these biorhythms provide an indication of positive and negative impact on your life in those areas. You can probably already recognize that there are days where your energy levels vary considerably.

SEASONAL AFFECTIVE DISORDER

Environmental aspects can impact on our lives. Consider the differences between the "winter blues", or seasonal affective disorder (SAD), and how you feel on a sunny day. SAD-affected individuals become anxious, irritable or depressed as light levels decrease in winter. There is a tendency to stop doing as much physical activity, which can directly affect energy levels. A well-recognized treatment is bright light therapy, which exposes an individual to bright-light for a period of time each day.

REDUCING ENERGY LEVELS

Some people may feel they need to rein in their energy at times. If you are a naturally exuberant person and sometimes overshadow others, try reducing your energy by changing your language to fit the situation. For example, words like "fun" might not sit comfortably with more serious individuals. Adopt a similar body language to the people you are with; sit back and watch how they act and subtly emulate them. Speak slowly and don't stay in a situation too long if your energy needs a different output. Find a way of releasing your energy elsewhere, then return afterwards if necessary.

WAYS TO AVOID SAD

- Be aware of your energy levels and how you feel.
- Go out on sunny winter days for as long as you can.
- Expose yourself to as much light as possible on overcast days.
- Keep physically active and eat healthily.
- Plan fun things to do and look forward to them.

LIFE PHASES AND ENERGY LEVELS

Our energy requirements vary enormously from birth to old age, and there are key times when our bodies have further challenges. For example, at puberty, there are physical changes, and the onset of puberty also encompasses psychological and cultural influences on adolescent energy levels.

PREGNANCY

This puts massive demands on the body. Many women feel exhausted during the first trimester and need to nap during the day. While the number of calories needed on a daily basis increases by about 300 towards the end of pregnancy, a pregnant woman has more need for nutrients like iron, calcium, protein and folic acid. As a woman moves into the second trimester, the benefits of staying active and eating healthily help her with the energy she needs for herself and her growing child.

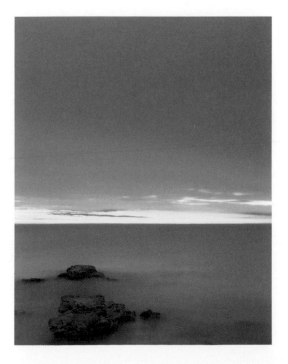

CHILDBIRTH

Giving birth puts a considerable strain on the mind, body and spirit. As well as the physical hardship of labour, there is also an emotional response to the hormones in the body. The energy expended to give birth can leave a woman feeling anything from exhausted to euphoric (or both), depending on her experience.

MENOPAUSE

The menopause generally refers to the time that comes immediately before, during and after the cessation of menstruation. The resulting hormonal changes affect many women. Diet, exercise and medication are thought to add to the symptoms and can have a severe impact on a woman's lifestyle. Reducing stress levels, exercising, eating healthily and reducing caffeine, smoking and alcohol, can all help.

AGE

Growing older can have a tremendous effect on energy levels. It may be that you discover new creative or intellectual energy as you move into your later years. Of course, physical changes that affect us as we age often have a major impact upon us, especially if we are limited by pain, illness or physical difficulties. It is also important to note that emotional problems can be just as draining and can affect us at any time. Many people welcome retirement as an opportunity for self-directed personal time with family and friends. For others, bridging the gap between a busy working life and no job to go to can be a challenge. Planning to meet your own needs is important.

YOUR PHYSICAL WELL-BEING

You can influence your own personal physical well-being through good nutrition, fitness and understanding your own health, whatever your age. This has a knock-on effect to your emotional and intellectual well-being, as well as having both short and long-term health benefits. The mind, body and soul are interlinked and as you improve your physical body, your brain will function more efficiently and you will find yourself able to cope more easily with the everyday stresses that 21st-century living brings.

WARNING SIGNALS

Our bodies provide us with a great deal of feedback if we just choose to stop and listen. Ask yourself the questions that follow. Make a note of your answers in a notebook. You might even want to spend a few days becoming aware of the messages your body is giving you and making changes to see what effect those changes have.

- Have you noticed changes in your energy as a result of what you eat and drink?

- What happens when you feel exhausted and eat unhealthy snacks?

- What happens when you give yourself some time for self-care and a balanced meal?

- Is your energy expenditure based on driving a car to work, or sitting in an office, or watching TV? Are you out taking regular walks?

- Are you listening to your warning signals, or do you tend to keep on going until you have overdone it?

The next page provides a list of warning signals. Tick any that you think apply to you. Add comments about how any relevant "red flags" make you feel and what triggers these warning signals. Make sure you do something to implement change. There are lots of tips and techniques throughout this book to help you on your way.

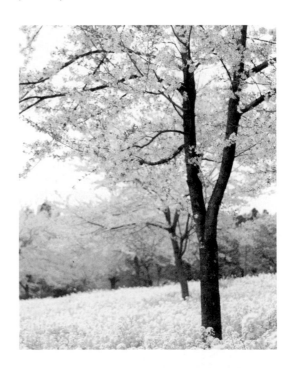

RED FLAGS

Physical

- ( ) Dehydration
- ( ) Over-indulgence
- ( ) Living off caffeine
- ( ) Over-use of sugar
- ( ) Lack of exercise
- ( ) Poor nutrition
- ( ) Lack of quality sleep

Emotional

- ( ) Focus on the negatives
- ( ) Living with fear
- ( ) Leaning on alcohol or cigarettes
- ( ) Mood swings
- ( ) Stress
- ( ) Living on a short fuse

Intellectual

- ( ) Poor memory
- ( ) Lack of concentration
- ( ) Imbalance in work, rest and play
- ( ) Poor diet
- ( ) Living in clutter
- ( ) Poor working environment
- ( ) Lack of stimulation of the brain

Personal

- ( ) Poorly defined values and beliefs
- ( ) Not living by those values and beliefs
- ( ) Work/life imbalance
- ( ) Poor relationships with colleagues
- ( ) Not being authentic to self
- ( ) Poor communication skills
- ( ) Lack of sexual energy
- ( ) Feeling drained

Spiritual

- ( ) Lack of purpose in life
- ( ) Negative habit patterns
- ( ) Poor self-esteem
- ( ) Mind, body and spirit imbalance
- ( ) Poor intuition
- ( ) Lack of empathy
- ( ) Lack of compassion

Creative

- ( ) Blocked creativity
- ( ) Lack of creative knowledge
- ( ) Poor goal-setting
- ( ) Inability to complete tasks
- ( ) Poor time management

ENERGY PROFILES

Do you find it difficult to get out of bed in the morning? Do you sometimes find yourself lacking in "get up and go" and wish you had more energy so you could do more with your life? Awareness of your own personal energy levels allows you to take control and initiate change. This section allows you to discover your own energy profile. Seeing your own personalized energy profile laid out on paper in front of you will provide you with all the necessary information to identify areas where you are lacking in energy and enable you to fulfil your potential. Remember that awareness is the key to action.

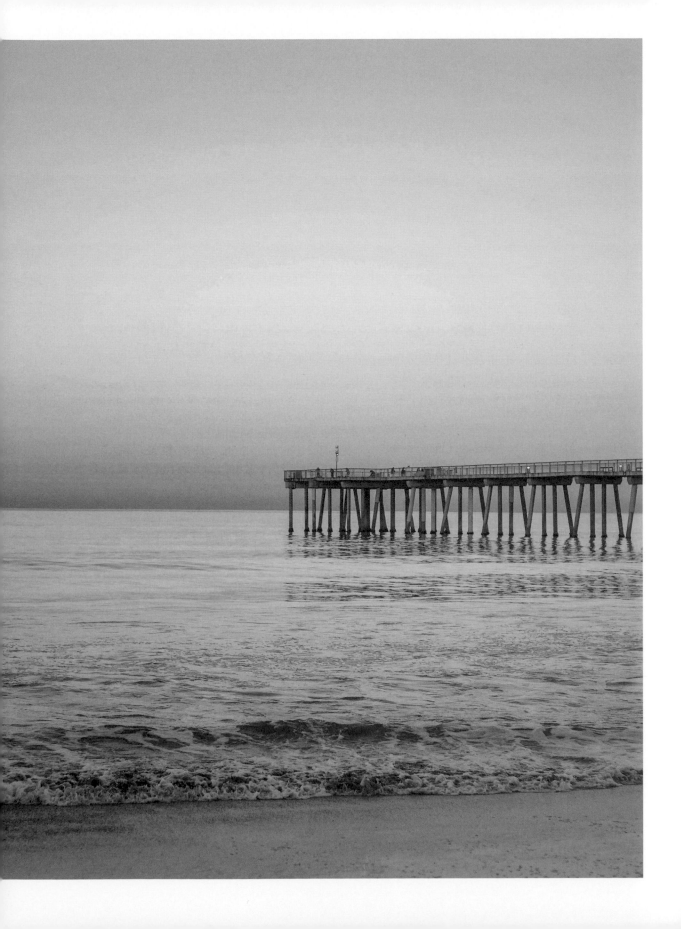

YOUR ENERGY PROFILE

This section allows you to discover your personal energy profile. The overall profile is split into the following six areas:

- Physical energy
- Emotional energy
- Intellectual energy
- Creative energy
- Personal energy
- Spiritual energy

ENERGY LEVELS

You can find your level in each of these six areas by answering a questionnaire, totalling your scores and reviewing your score against the corresponding profiles.

Note: Some people consider that they are so firmly rooted in the material world that they don't feel they have a spiritual aspect. To that end, there are three additional questions at the end of the questionnaire, which directly refer to spirituality; the other seven questions are taken from across the profiles. Just miss out this section if it is one that you don't consider to be relevant to you.

STEP-BY-STEP GUIDE

1 Answer the questionnaire on pages 26–29.
2 Move to the physical energy profile and total your scores as instructed.
3 Read the profile that matches your score.
4 Complete for all profiles.

INTERPRETING YOUR PROFILE

Once you have scored all of your energy profiles, it is time to put it together. Write the summary of your scores in the grid on page 43 and then plot each profile within the ring. You can even colour it in, in a similar way to the example, if you choose (if you do, you may find you scored highly on creative energy!).

ACTING ON IT

Now you should have a complete energy profile to stick on your wall or fridge. How balanced are you? Are you happy with your strengths and where they lie? If not, then what are you going do about it?

One approach is to take the energy profile where you feel you need the most improvement and to move straight to the techniques section and read the relevant pages. You may find the planning tool and checklist on pages 122–123 useful to help you do this in a structured way. However you choose to start improving your energy levels, my main piece of advice is just give it a go, right now, and don't put it off until tomorrow or next week.

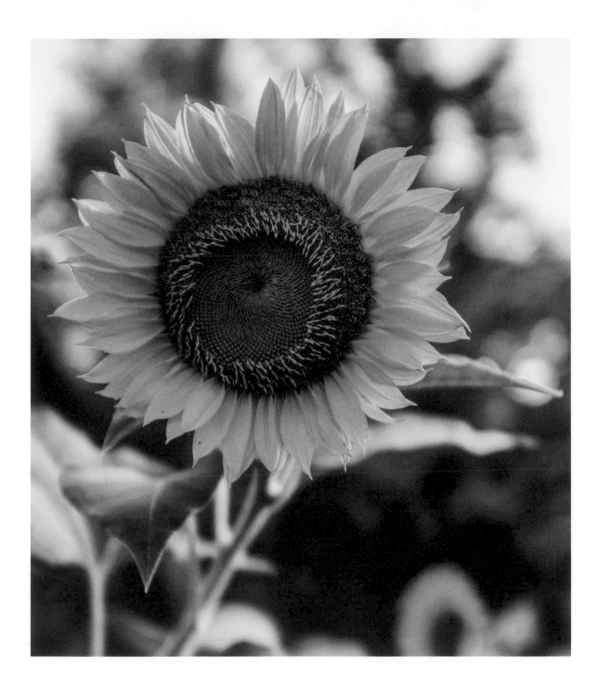

REVIEWING YOUR PROGRESS

It is a good idea to keep the first overall energy profile sheet you draw up as you can come back and answer the questions again in a few weeks' or months' time and compare the two.

You could even draw your goals on the sheet to give you something to work towards. There are many tools to help you on your way to a more energized you. Use as many as you can.

QUESTIONNAIRE

Don't think for too long about your answers and be honest with yourself about how you are, rather than how you would like to be. The questionnaire is not a standardized test, but a way of getting you to think about yourself.

1 I can concentrate for long stretches of time without allowing myself to be distracted

DISAGREE	0	1	2	3	4	5	AGREE

2 I enjoy visualizing the future

DISAGREE	0	1	2	3	4	5	AGREE

3 I eat healthily

DISAGREE	0	1	2	3	4	5	AGREE

4 I love being with friends more than I love solitude

DISAGREE	0	1	2	3	4	5	AGREE

5 I hold very strong beliefs

DISAGREE	0	1	2	3	4	5	AGREE

6 I love to discover new ideas

DISAGREE	0	1	2	3	4	5	AGREE

7 I use stories to make my point when I talk to people

DISAGREE	0	1	2	3	4	5	AGREE

8 I am full of physical energy

DISAGREE	0	1	2	3	4	5	AGREE

9 I am never lonely

DISAGREE	0	1	2	3	4	5	AGREE

10 Values are important to me

DISAGREE	0	1	2	3	4	5	AGREE

11 I am good at thinking, creating and problem-solving

DISAGREE | 0 | 1 | 2 | 3 | 4 | 5 | AGREE

12 I love to make up stories in my head

DISAGREE | 0 | 1 | 2 | 3 | 4 | 5 | AGREE

13 I never have trouble getting out of bed in the morning

DISAGREE | 0 | 1 | 2 | 3 | 4 | 5 | AGREE

14 I manage to control emotions of hatred and anger

DISAGREE | 0 | 1 | 2 | 3 | 4 | 5 | AGREE

15 I never procrastinate

DISAGREE | 0 | 1 | 2 | 3 | 4 | 5 | AGREE

16 Coming up with new ideas and abilities is exciting

DISAGREE | 0 | 1 | 2 | 3 | 4 | 5 | AGREE

17 I welcome the idea of being successfully creative

DISAGREE | 0 | 1 | 2 | 3 | 4 | 5 | AGREE

18 I exercise at least three times a week

DISAGREE | 0 | 1 | 2 | 3 | 4 | 5 | AGREE

19 Friendship is important to me

DISAGREE | 0 | 1 | 2 | 3 | 4 | 5 | AGREE

20 It is nice to be liked, but not necessary

DISAGREE | 0 | 1 | 2 | 3 | 4 | 5 | AGREE

21 I like to keep my mind razor-sharp

DISAGREE | 0 | 1 | 2 | 3 | 4 | 5 | AGREE

22 I am able to see new things through

DISAGREE | 0 | 1 | 2 | 3 | 4 | 5 | AGREE

23 Physical activity is one of my favourite things

DISAGREE | 0 | 1 | 2 | 3 | 4 | 5 | AGREE

24 I like to be part of activities that involve my friends

DISAGREE | 0 | 1 | 2 | 3 | 4 | 5 | AGREE

25 I am very self-confident in most situations

DISAGREE | 0 | 1 | 2 | 3 | 4 | 5 | AGREE

26 I am always reading at least one book or occupied by an intellectual activity

DISAGREE | 0 | 1 | 2 | 3 | 4 | 5 | AGREE

27 I love to be stimulated by the creativity of others

DISAGREE | 0 | 1 | 2 | 3 | 4 | 5 | AGREE

28 I don't like being a couch potato

DISAGREE | 0 | 1 | 2 | 3 | 4 | 5 | AGREE

29 Most people like me immediately

DISAGREE | 0 | 1 | 2 | 3 | 4 | 5 | AGREE

30 What people think of me is unimportant

DISAGREE | 0 | 1 | 2 | 3 | 4 | 5 | AGREE

31 I would rather have an original, useful idea than most other things

DISAGREE | 0 | 1 | 2 | 3 | 4 | 5 | AGREE

32 When I listen to good music, I feel inspired

DISAGREE | 0 | 1 | 2 | 3 | 4 | 5 | AGREE

33 My friends often ask me where I get my energy from

DISAGREE | 0 | 1 | 2 | 3 | 4 | 5 | AGREE

34 I respect the beliefs of others

DISAGREE | 0 | 1 | 2 | 3 | 4 | 5 | AGREE

35 By my own standards, I am very successful

DISAGREE | 0 | 1 | 2 | 3 | 4 | 5 | AGREE

36 I would like to be known for my ideas rather than any other part of my character

DISAGREE | 0 | 1 | 2 | 3 | 4 | 5 | AGREE

37 My friends think I am creative

DISAGREE | 0 | 1 | 2 | 3 | 4 | 5 | AGREE

38 I recover quickly from a lack of sleep

DISAGREE | 0 | 1 | 2 | 3 | 4 | 5 | AGREE

39 I am sensitive to the feelings of others

DISAGREE | 0 | 1 | 2 | 3 | 4 | 5 | AGREE

40 I am unconventional

DISAGREE | 0 | 1 | 2 | 3 | 4 | 5 | AGREE

41 People admire my intellect

DISAGREE | 0 | 1 | 2 | 3 | 4 | 5 | AGREE

42 I am a creative person

DISAGREE | 0 | 1 | 2 | 3 | 4 | 5 | AGREE

43 My bodyweight is just about perfect

DISAGREE | 0 | 1 | 2 | 3 | 4 | 5 | AGREE

44 I encourage shy people to join in

DISAGREE | 0 | 1 | 2 | 3 | 4 | 5 | AGREE

45 I know what motivates me

DISAGREE | 0 | 1 | 2 | 3 | 4 | 5 | AGREE

46 I have a powerful intellect

DISAGREE | 0 | 1 | 2 | 3 | 4 | 5 | AGREE

47 I am always coming up with new ideas

DISAGREE | 0 | 1 | 2 | 3 | 4 | 5 | AGREE

48 I pay attention to my physical condition

DISAGREE | 0 | 1 | 2 | 3 | 4 | 5 | AGREE

49 Love is important to me

DISAGREE | 0 | 1 | 2 | 3 | 4 | 5 | AGREE

50 I know what my purpose in life is

DISAGREE | 0 | 1 | 2 | 3 | 4 | 5 | AGREE

51 I think of myself as a spiritual person

DISAGREE | 0 | 1 | 2 | 3 | 4 | 5 | AGREE

52 I believe in the importance of spirituality

DISAGREE | 0 | 1 | 2 | 3 | 4 | 5 | AGREE

53 I have beliefs beyond the worldly and the immediate

DISAGREE | 0 | 1 | 2 | 3 | 4 | 5 | AGREE

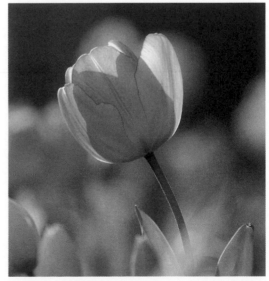

YOUR PHYSICAL PROFILE

Total your scores to questions 3, 8, 13, 18, 23, 28, 33, 38, 43 and 48 in the questionnaire and plot your physical energy profile on page 43. Once you have done this, find your corresponding level below and read your personal physical energy profile.

QUESTION	3	8	13	18	23	28	33	38	43	48	TOTAL
YOUR SCORE											

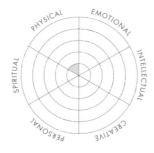

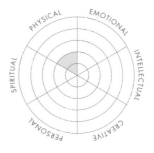

0–10

You have extremely low levels of physical energy and would benefit from many techniques in this book; in fact, they could change your whole outlook on life. It would be worthwhile visiting your doctor to rule out any health problems; otherwise, your low score is an urgent wake-up call and you need to move straight on to the techniques and give yourself a goal of adopting the dietary habits (see pages 50–51) within a month.

• The advice on Energy angels and vampires on pages 106–107 will give you an insight into people who would help and support you or hinder and stop your progress.

11–20

You have very low levels of physical energy. This low level could have been caused by many factors in your life. Your body is an integral part of a system that includes your thinking, feelings and moods. You need to work on all aspects of your energy, because they all affect physical well-being. A big boost in one area of your life could be just the thing your body needs to feel more energized physically. This boost could be getting the best exercise and dietary advice and to make sure you at least do all of the physical techniques (see pages 48–59) in this book.

• See also the technique on Connecting mind, body and spirit on page 110.

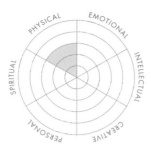

21–30

Your energy levels are mid-range. There are probably times when you feel full of energy and others when you wish you had more. Your physical energy is dependent on your energy as a whole, so ask yourself if anything is out of step in your life. Bring balance into everything you do. Don't forget the importance of quality rest and nutrition. Think of the food and drink that enters your body today as forming your body – and its energy levels – tomorrow. In parallel, think about finding a form of exercise you enjoy and do it regularly. Slowly but surely, your energy will increase. To accelerate the process, tell yourself that you are already full of energy and think it often.

• Try using the Visualization exercises on pages 94–95 and 118–119 to imagine yourself healthier, brighter and more energetic.

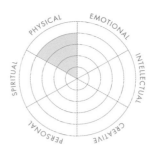

31–40

You have an excellent basis of fitness and health. It may be that you could feel even better if you were a little more consistent in your exercise and eating habits. Remember that you have a right to feel as great as possible. Build your health and fitness regime into your life. If family and friends occasionally have to take a back seat that is fine, as they will get far more from you when you have maximized your physical energy.

• The technique of Achieving goals on page 88 might be appropriate at this stage.

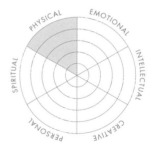

41–50

You are bouncing with physical energy and in the best of health. You know how to achieve physical fitness, so you are able to go about achieving in other areas of your life. Physical fitness is not one more barrier that you have to overcome – it is an asset to support your achievement of everything you want in life.

• Take time to look through the Physical techniques on pages 48–59, as there just might be something there that you have not yet tried!

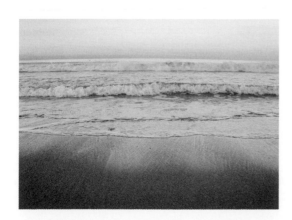

YOUR EMOTIONAL PROFILE

Total your scores to questions 4, 9, 14, 19, 24, 29, 34, 39, 44 and 49 in the questionnaire and plot your emotional energy profile on page 43. Once you have done this, find your corresponding level below and read your personal emotional energy profile.

QUESTION	4	9	14	19	24	29	34	39	44	49	TOTAL
YOUR SCORE											

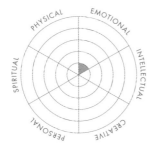

0–10

You have extremely low levels of emotional energy and you would benefit from using many of the techniques in this book; in fact, they could help you change your attitude to how you live your life. Stop and consider for a moment whether your score is based on some underlying issues for which you might benefit from professional help. If so, then why not take this as a nudge and get support now? Otherwise, read the strategies for gaining positive emotional energy on page 63.

• The advice on Energy angels and vampires on pages 106–107 will give you an insight into people who would help or hinder you in your progress.

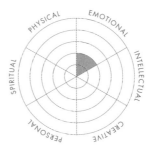

11–20

You have very low levels of emotional energy which could have been caused by influences in your life going back many years. You could be living or working with an energy vampire who is draining you emotionally. You may find it difficult to be in social groups, or have problems with giving out love. Whatever your reasons are, remember that you get back what you give out. So try giving out some love and understanding and wait for it to flood back to you, and search out some energy angels (see page 106) to help replenish you while you learn the habits to do it on your own.

• See also the Physical energy techniques on pages 48–59, which will give you the strength and physical energy to focus.

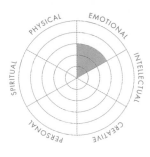

21–30

Your emotional levels are mid-range. The best advice is to learn to love and value yourself. You have as much right to happiness as anyone else, and it is just out there waiting for you. You don't have to have a smile plastered on your face for 24 hours a day, and you don't need to be the life and soul of the party. You just need to recognize your own worth and quietly go about life making sure that you use all your talents to the best of your abilities. Be true to yourself and others will sense that you are genuine, and they will give their emotional energy to you in bucket loads.

• You may find the section on Meditation on pages 116–117 helpful.

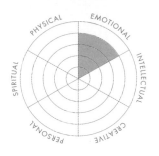

31–40

You have a well-balanced personality that respects and is sensitive to the needs of people, but does not cross the line into unwanted interference in the lives of others. Don't be scared of being unconventional sometimes – if that is what is required. Use your ability to get on well with people to help both them and yourself. Go out of your way to make other people feel special and successful – it will always come back to you.

• Have a read of the Personal energy tips on page 97 to add to your positive energy.

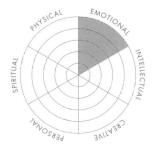

41–50

You are a larger-than-life character who gets noticed. You are also part of a tiny percentage of the population, because people who are both socially extrovert and very sensitive to the needs and feelings of others are rare. Either that, or you have a biased view of yourself! Carry on enjoying life, giving pleasure to others and taking

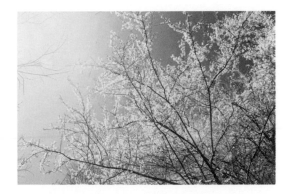

happiness where you can find it. Just make sure that you use the appropriate energy at the appropriate times.

• Take time to look through the Emotional techniques on pages 60–71, as you may find something useful in there.

YOUR INTELLECTUAL PROFILE

Total your scores to questions 1, 6, 11, 16, 21, 26, 31, 36, 41 and 46 in the questionnaire and plot your intellectual energy profile on page 43. Once you have done this, find your corresponding level below and read your personal intellectual energy profile.

QUESTION	1	6	11	16	21	26	31	36	41	46	TOTAL
YOUR SCORE											

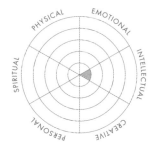

0–10

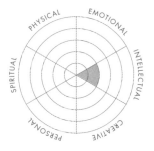

11–20

You have extremely low levels of intellectual energy. Don't worry, however, as there are many ways to train the brain. The first step is starting to believe in your intellectual self and to begin doing something to improve your energy levels in this area.

• You will find the Stimulating the brain section on pages 80–83 an excellent place to start, and you should aim to set yourself a goal of doing one or more of these activities each day. You will soon notice massive changes in your energy levels.

You have very low levels of intellectual energy. Without looking into new ideas, you are unlikely to come up with any of your own. You are missing out greatly on one of the great spices of life! It is also possible that you under-rate your intellectual capabilities. Remember a time when your thinking has produced a new way of doing things, even if it is only a minor achievement. Use that memory to motivate your thinking in the future. Most of all, you should develop your powers of concentration; this needs practice and application. Take a subject you are interested in and resolve to become an expert in it.

• See also the technique on Motivation on page 55; although it is based on physical energy, many of the factors are relevant.

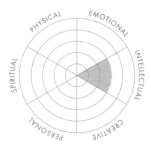

21–30

Your intellectual energy is mid-range, but may be balanced by scores in other areas. Work on improving concentration and realize that without new knowledge new ideas are more difficult to generate, and ideas are the engines of change. If you want to change, you must sharpen your concentration and apply your knowledge at every opportunity.

• Make sure your diet is healthy and you have sufficient rest. A healthy diet on page 50–51 leads to a healthier brain.

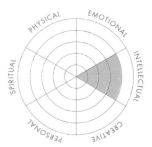

31–40

You have good intellectual energy, and have a very healthy love of thinking and new ideas. The knowledge you acquire through your intellectual pursuits will enable you to remain flexible, skilled and interesting, and you will be able to adapt to shifting circumstances. You can also work on your self-discipline, by setting yourself targets and adopting good habits.

• You may find the How to relieve a stressful situation technique on page 71 useful.

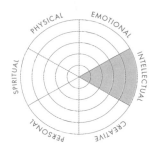

41–50

You have excellent intellectual energy. For you, ideas are not work – they are play. Your love of intellectual pursuits and new ideas will always mean that you are interesting and adaptable to change. You may be a great inventor, artist or philosopher, depending on your other results. However, it is possible that your love for the life of the mind makes you seem a bit cold and separate to others, so you may need to work on your emotional intelligence. Is your self-confidence when it comes to ideas reflected by your confidence in social situations? Remember that it is all about balance.

• Consider how well you manage your emotional strengths by scoring yourself on the Emotional strategies on page 63.

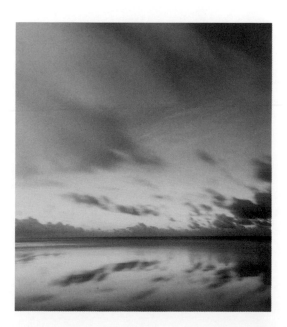

YOUR CREATIVE PROFILE

Total your scores to questions 2, 7, 12, 17, 22, 27, 32, 37, 42 and 47 in the questionnaire and plot your creative energy profile on page 43. Once you have done this, find your corresponding level below and read your own personal creative energy profile.

QUESTION	2	7	12	17	22	27	32	37	42	47	TOTAL
YOUR SCORE											

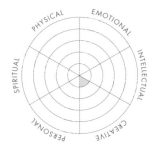

0–10

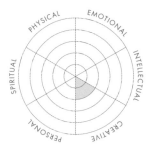

11–20

You have extremely low levels of creative energy. Perhaps you are one of those people who switch off when they hear the word "creative". If so, then ask yourself what it is about the word that you don't like. There are very few uncreative people in this world; just look around you to see how ideas, products and artistic objects are abundant. There are many ways of being creative – perhaps you don't believe yourself to be creative and are blocked.

• You will find the section on Dealing with blockages on page 92 a good starting point to unleash your creative energy. If you feel panicky about the word "creative", read Dealing with stress on pages 70–71.

You have very low levels of creative energy and are not using two of the most powerful tools at your disposal – imagination and visualization. Use your imagination to bring the future you want into existence; otherwise you may end up with a future you don't want. Then use visualization to fill in the details of exactly how things will be. Creative use of the imagination is not just about the future; it is about living a wonderful life today. Have a go at the exercises in the creative energy techniques section on pages 84–95 – you will be amazed at the results.

• There are some useful Visualization exercises on pages 94–95.

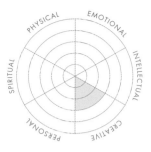

21–30

Your creative energy is mid-range. Set yourself some goals and then practise the different suggestions given in the creative energy techniques section (see pages 84–95). Be aware that this is not just about "artistic" creativity; it is about creating the future for yourself that you want and getting on and achieving your goals. Before you use visualization techniques, always find some meditative silence first. You need to be calm, quiet and comfortable when you are preparing to get the creative juices flowing.

• You will find further Visualization techniques on pages 118–119.

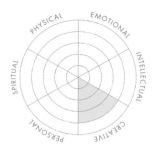

31–40

You have good creative energy, and you are well on your way to bringing the life that you want into existence. Have confidence in your ability to do so, as creating your own life is the most important act of imagination that anyone can do. Make sure that you find time to have an outlet for your artistic and creative energies; if not, frustration may result. How you manage your time will have a major influence on your ability to use your creative energy to good effect.

• The Work/life balance section on page 98 looks at how you can marry different roles and responsibilities together.

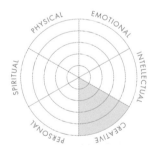

41–50

You have excellent creative energy. You are imaginative, creative and artistic. You see your own life for the work of art that it is – something entirely under your control, like a painter's canvas. It is important that you don't "hide your light under a bushel"; find a worthy outlet for your imagination that will make a difference in

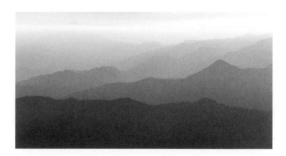

the world. It is hard to find any words of caution for the truly imaginative, other than to say that you should be sure to marry your creative abilities to your values and beliefs, and keep them in balance with your other energy profiles.

• Make sure you read the Creative techniques section on pages 84–95 as it may create some more ideas.

YOUR PERSONAL PROFILE

Total your scores to questions 5, 10, 15, 20, 25, 30, 35, 40, 45 and 50 in the questionnaire and plot your personal energy profile on page 43. Once you have done this, find your corresponding level below and read your personal energy profile.

QUESTION	5	10	15	20	25	30	35	40	45	50	TOTAL
YOUR SCORE											

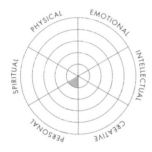

0–10

You have extremely low levels of personal energy, which may be due to a feeling of low self-esteem. Personal energy is about how you feel about yourself. Is this a true representation or are you self-critical? Whatever the answer, it is essential that you do something to improve your view of yourself, as this will have a major impact on your enjoyment of life and ability to be successful. Work through the personal energy techniques section and consider the life phase you are in currently and where you would like your personal energy to be.

• You may find the section on Connecting mind, body and spirit on page 110 useful to give you a holistic grounding.

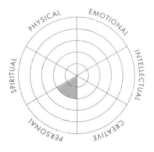

11–20

You have very low levels of personal energy. It is likely that you have several areas of your life where you are under-performing. There may be issues with your outlook on life that makes each other worse. It is a vicious circle – your lack of direction may lead to a lack of self-confidence, causing you not to develop strong values and beliefs that you need for motivation and direction. Improvement in one of these areas will have a knock-on effect on the others. Soon, with a little willpower, determination and visualization, you can be in a positive-feedback situation where things quickly get better – a virtuous circle!

• See the Vicious and Virtuous energy cycles on page 52 in relation to drinks.

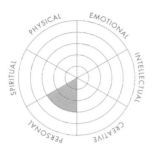

21–30

Your energy levels are mid-range. Make it your mission to get things done. Realize that the reason you are not getting things done may be due to your own lack of self-confidence. So, before undertaking something you have been avoiding, visualize a past success. Amplify that image of your successful self – make it brighter, more colourful, more beautiful. That is the capable you – the you who is going to take the next difficult thing that comes along by the scruff of the neck. Build on it, one success at a time.

• See the Healthy diet section on pages 50–51 for advice that will help your energy levels in all areas of your profile.

31–40

You have high levels of personal energy. You are self-confident, successful and motivated. You seem to have a superb moral balance in your life between what is important internally and externally. You know what you want and you are going to get it, but would probably be horrified to get success at someone else's expense. You have strong values that help you to make decisions instinctively, and without regret. You are an energy angel (see page 106).

• Following the principles in Creating the right physical environment on pages 78–79 will have a knock-on effect on your ability to keep your energy levels raised and recharged.

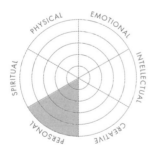

41–50

You have excellent levels of personal energy. Your self-confidence and independence is inspiring. This can bring you success or unhappiness. As every strength is our weakness, so might your single-mindedness come across as inflexibility, self-confidence as arrogance and self-reliance

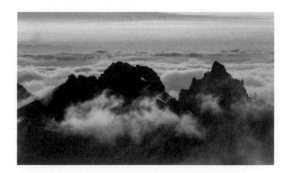

as contempt. Be aware of this and keep your personal energy levels in check. There is a fine line between an energy angel and an energy vampire (see pages 106–107). It is in your hands.

• You may find the Achieve your goals section on page 88 helpful.

YOUR SPIRITUAL PROFILE

Total your scores to questions 2, 5, 9, 10, 30, 34, 50, 51, 52 and 53 in the questionnaire and plot your spiritual energy profile on page 43. Once you have done this, find your corresponding level below and read your personal spiritual energy profile.

QUESTION	2	5	9	10	30	34	50	51	52	53	TOTAL
YOUR SCORE											

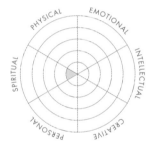

0–10

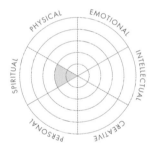

11–20

You have extremely low levels of spiritual energy and may not see yourself as a spiritual being. If this is by choice, this is fine. If this is not the case, and you do consider yourself a spiritual person, then you will find a significant transformation in your life if you use the exercises in the spiritual energy techniques section (see pages 108–119) to help you unblock your energy channels. There may be other elements holding you back from pursuing your dreams, so think about whether you need to balance or improve your other energies first.

• Why not flick through the contents of this book to see which energy technique calls out to you, and incorporate it into your life right now?

You have very low levels of spiritual energy. Again, this may be by choice. If spirituality is important to you, then adopting the strategies to connect your mind, body and spirit will be a springboard that will take you onto a new plane of existence.

• You may find that the Complementary energizers on page 114–115 will help give you the energy needed to take the next step to finding a spiritually energized you.

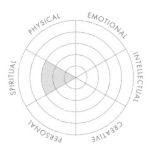

21–30

Your spiritual energy levels are mid-range and spirituality is probably one of those things that you can sense, but does not have any tangible meaning to you. It may be that you are too busy with other aspects of your life to be able to focus on it at the moment. As you become ready to explore this part of your nature, you will find the spiritual doors will open. If you want to accelerate this, try using the visualization techniques on pages 118–119 to picture the "you" that you want to become.

• If you have not read it already, look at Energy around the world on pages 10–13 for some inspirational methods – see what attracts you and research it further.

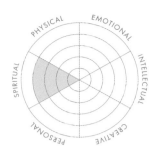

31–40

You have high levels of spiritual energy and probably have a well-developed intuition and sense of yourself in connection with a greater energy. This will bring you a peace, sense of connectedness and ability to be compassionate and non-judgemental to others. Treating others as you would like to be treated is probably of importance to you, as is feeling that you are fair and just. However you feel within, there is still so much to learn in the world, and to improve on. Take time to go through the techniques, even if you already have something similar in your life; there might be something there waiting specifically for you.

• Creativity can be an good for stimulating spirituality. See Stimulate your creativity on pages 86–87.

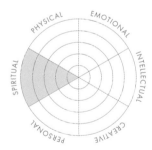

41–50

You have extremely high levels of spiritual energy and see yourself as very spiritual. Most people probably find you a calming influence and think of you as a bit of a Mother Teresa. However, you may have a tendency to take this slightly too far; some may find your views a bit "out there" or

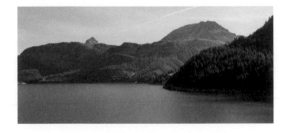

plain annoying. Remember that these are your views, which can vary from others, and who is to say which viewpoint is better? Be who you choose to be and live by your values and beliefs.

• You may find the Emotional strategies on pages 60–63 useful to read through as a check on your own spiritual balance.

YOUR OVERALL PROFILE

It is now time to put your profile together. As you worked through the profiles in the earlier sections, you may have filled out the grid on the following page; if not, then do so now. If you don't want to write in the book, use a copy; then you can use it again for reviewing your changes. You should have something that looks like this example:

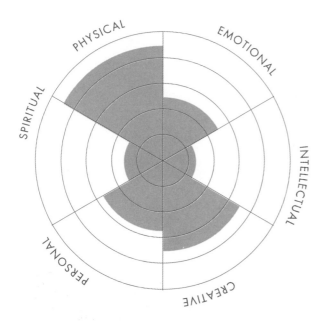

EXAMPLE ENERGY GRID

PHYSICAL ENERGY	46
EMOTIONAL ENERGY	24
INTELLECTUAL ENERGY	12
CREATIVE ENERGY	35
PERSONAL ENERGY	27
SPIRITUAL ENERGY	13

Now fill in your energy profile on the circular diagram and look at its shape. Each concentric ring represents 10 points, and there is a maximum score of 50. So, if you have scored 25, colour in up to the middle of the third band. (If you have chosen not to fill in the spiritual energy profile, overlap the physical and creative profiles so that you don't have any gaps.) Imagine this is your energy wheel.

How in balance is it? It may be that you need more energy in certain areas – it is up to you to decide what you need so that you can achieve the balance to meet your needs. It also may be important to use more energy at different times depending on what is going on in your life. Remember that most people need a minimum of a mid-range score in each area so you have the resource to call on if you need it.

YOUR ENERGY GRID

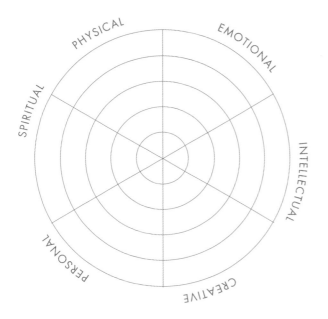

PHYSICAL ENERGY

EMOTIONAL ENERGY

INTELLECTUAL ENERGY

CREATIVE ENERGY

PERSONAL ENERGY

SPIRITUAL ENERGY

Put your overall profile somewhere you can see it every day. You might want to date it and use similar colours to the profile above. You will find this useful for comparison later when you measure your success by completing the questionnaire again.

After completing your overall energy profile, go to the techniques section to find theory, tips and strategies to increase your energy levels where you need it most. Work on balancing your energy wheel to suit you! Find the area that is the weakest and concentrate on improving your energy in that area first. Set yourself a realistic goal and then work on improving each area. You are your own energy source.

EXTRA ENERGY FACTORS

Well done, you have now completed your overall energy profile. However, as usual in life, nothing is quite that simple. To truly personalize your energy profile, you need to take into account the complexities that make you the unique and incredible person you are, as well as lifestyle factors that affect your energy levels.

STRENGTHS AND WEAKNESSES

Each of the profiles is based on a series of questions. There are only so many questions that can be asked in the space of a single book covering such a vast subject. For example, your score may be mid-range, but actually you may have marked yourself high on some questions and low on others.

Take a moment now to reflect on each profile (go back and read the questions again if necessary with their corresponding scores) and identify whether there are any particular strengths or weaknesses. If you know how, you could even make it into a "strengths, weaknesses, opportunities and threats" (SWOT) analysis. Either use the table or use a creative brainstorming diagram (like the example shown) to elicit your thoughts and feelings and therefore analyse yourself one step further.

BRAINSTORMING DIAGRAM

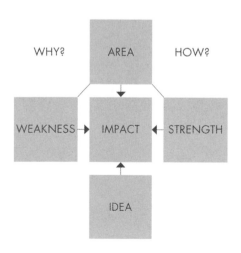

ENERGY TYPE	STRENGTHS	WEAKNESSES
PHYSICAL ENERGY		
EMOTIONAL ENERGY		
INTELLECTUAL ENERGY		
CREATIVE ENERGY		
PERSONAL ENERGY		
SPIRITUAL ENERGY		

CONSTRAINTS

The second issue is those extra factors that we cannot do much about, but need to work with. It would be fun to focus on ourselves and our energy levels for as long as we need to and to the exclusion of all else. However, most of us have responsibilities in our lives including the need to earn money to live, eat and socialize. A few examples of the sorts of constraints we are under are included here. Put a tick beside the ones that apply to you and add any more you can think of. Add this list to your energy profile on the fridge door. Be proud of your commitments. This is about working within the constraints of life.

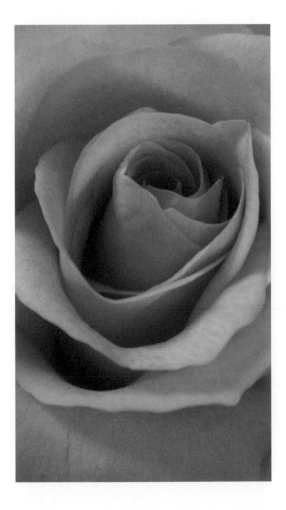

EVERYDAY CONSTRAINTS

○ **Children** – lack of sleep is a common issue in families with young children but older children and teenagers can also be demanding on your time and energy.

○ **Illness** – from the common cold to more severe diseases, all illnesses affect our energy levels. It is important to adjust activity levels to take account of physical symptoms.

○ **Insomnia** – whether having difficulty falling asleep or waking often in the night, a lack of sleep is probably the most important energy block.

○ **Obesity** – when the energy intake through food and drink exceeds energy expenditure, the excess energy is stored as fat. An obese person needs more physical energy to move around and can be more susceptible to certain diseases.

○ **Shift patterns** – many people work shift patterns and suffer a similar effect to jet lag but on a long-term basis.

○ **Travelling between time zones** – disrupts your body clock. The human body clock is designed to fit in with circadian rhythms, guiding us to times to fall asleep, wake up and eat meals. As time zones change, our internal body clock has to "catch up", which is commonly known as jet lag.

○ **Work** – most of us have to work to pay bills and earn money for extras in life. However, not all of us are in a job we love and the pressure of our responsibilities means that sometimes our jobs just need doing.

ENERGY
TECHNIQUES

This section is split into six parts: physical, emotional, intellectual, creative, personal and spiritual. Each part includes 12 pages of key techniques to help raise your energy level in that area. However, remember that energy is something that should always be in balance; so, even if your energy-level requirements are mainly physical you may still need to use techniques from other areas as well, as depletion of energy in one area may affect another.

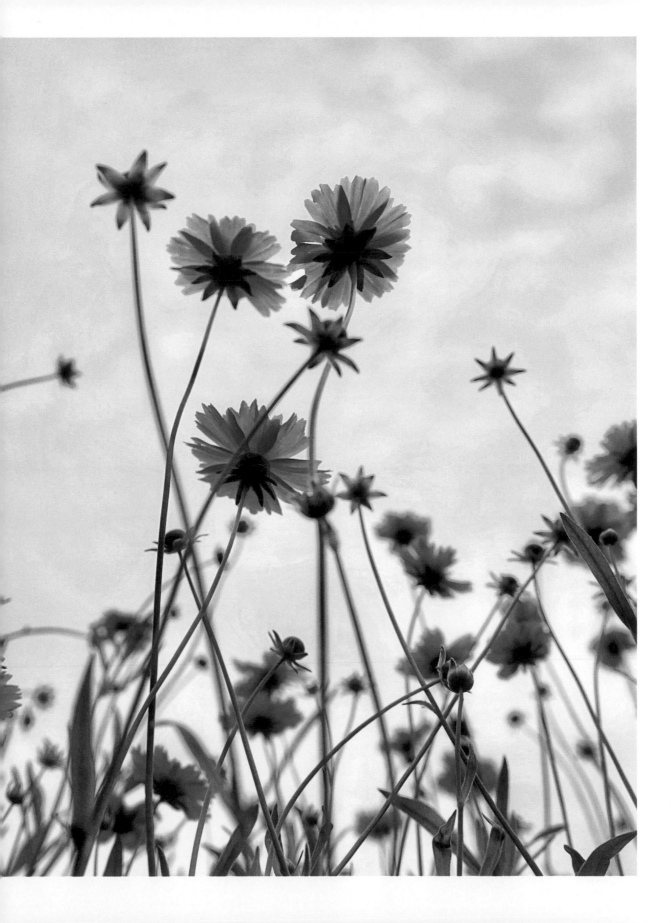

PHYSICAL TECHNIQUES

Physical energy comes from physical health, good nutrition and appropriate levels of exercise, as well as psychological and environmental aspects. Lack of physical activity increases the risk of mortality and diseases such as coronary heart disease, high blood pressure and depression. A well-known recommendation is for an individual to exercise aerobically for 30 minutes per day for a minimum of three days a week.

THE ENERGY EQUATION

Losing, gaining or maintaining weight is all about understanding how energy works in your body. You take energy in by eating and drinking and expend energy by normal metabolic means and daily activities. This means that, even when you lie in bed, you still use energy to function, but every extra bit of exercise you do uses more. To lose weight you need to use more calories than you put into your body, and to gain weight you need to consume more calories than you use.

Each of us have different calorific demands, which depends on our age, activity level and metabolism. Calories contain different nutritional benefits and having a balanced diet is important. Choose nutrient-rich, low-calorie foods and mix the different food groups. Make sure that you have lots of fruit and vegetables in your diet as well as a mix of proteins and complex carbohydrates. It is not just eating the right stuff, but ensuring that your body can absorb the nutrients it needs. Without the appropriate digestive enzymes, the nutrients remain locked in the food rather than passing into your bloodstream.

BODY MASS INDEX (BMI)

A well-recognized way of finding out if you are a healthy weight is through the body mass index (BMI) – but remember that your musculature will affect your results, so take this into account. The BMI is defined as your weight in kilograms divided by your height in metres squared:

$$BMI = kg / m^2$$

If you know your weight in pounds or stone, you might prefer one of these alternative equations:

$$BMI = 6.35 \times weight \text{ (stone)} / m^2$$
$$BMI = 703 \times weight \text{ (lb)} / in^2$$

BMI	CATEGORY
Less than 18.5	Underweight
18.5–25	Normal
25–30	Overweight
Over 30	Obese

ENERGY EXPENDITURE

EXAMPLE ACTIVITIES	ENERGY EXPENDED IN 30 MINUTES (AVERAGE MALE)	ENERGY EXPENDED IN 30 MINUTES (AVERAGE FEMALE)
Watching TV	39 calories	32 calories
Moderate sexual activity	50 calories	41 calories
General house cleaning	116 calories	95 calories
Walking to work	154 calories	127 calories
Dancing	173 calories	143 calories
Swimming	231 calories	191 calories
Running	308 calories	254 calories
Gardening	154 calories	127 calories

KEEP FIT

Being fit is more important than weight. If you focus on long-term physical fitness, this will have a major impact on your long-term energy levels, whatever your weight.

We expend less physical energy compared with our ancestors, but in an evolutionary sense our bodies have yet to catch up with these changes. Our grandparents expected to wash clothes by hand, grow their own vegetables and walk to the shops daily. Our bodies are suffering from the ease of eating fast food and the issues that technological living bring. There is no need to do anything complicated to lose weight, just be sensible and do things in moderation.

Choose the most nutritionally rich foods you can from each food group – those packed with vitamins, minerals, fibre and other nutrients, but lower in calories. Pick foods like fruits, vegetables, wholegrain, and fat-free or low-fat milk and milk products. A good maxim here is "Eat more wisely, rather than less".

LIFESTYLE

We all want different things from life and make different choices. One person's idea of pleasure may be another's penance. If you don't like the gym, don't go, but find other enjoyable ways of expending energy. Make high physical energy levels part of your everyday life.

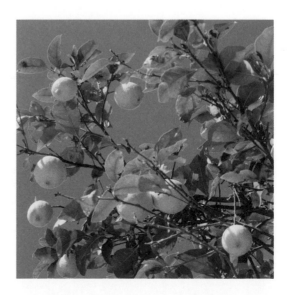

A HEALTHY DIET

There are many books on diets and different food fads, and there is not enough space here to begin to discuss them all. Instead, this section is about adopting basic eating habits, which will make a major difference to your energy levels and those of your family.

EAT A HEALTHY BREAKFAST

- Burn more calories during the day than if you had skipped breakfast.
- Your brain works better.
- Successful slimmers always eat breakfast.

EAT LITTLE AND OFTEN

(5–6 small meals/snacks a day)

- Smaller portions help stop over-eating.
- Keep your blood-sugar levels stable.
- Decrease cravings and mood swings.
- A big meal in the evening will disrupt sleep and you are less likely to burn off calories.

AVOID REFINED SUGARS

- They are addictive and can affect mood and energy.
- They are toxic to the body.
- They use up your body's stores of nutrients.

MODERATE CAFFEINE INTAKE

- It stimulates the central nervous system.
- It is addictive.
- Some people suffer withdrawal symptoms.

RECOGNIZE HUNGER SIGNALS

- Our wish to eat is often based on a psychological need.
- Start eating when you recognize your physical hunger signals.
- Eat slowly and savour your food.
- Stop when you are comfortably full.

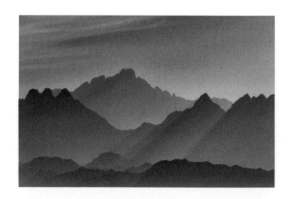

DRINK EIGHT GLASSES OF WATER A DAY

(around 2 litres (3½ pints))

• It improves your memory, concentration and energy levels.

• On average, 60 per cent of your bodyweight is water.

• Even mild dehydration can sap energy.

• The kidneys need water to function properly.

• Water contains no calories or fat.

EAT HIGH-ENERGY FOODS

• Beans and lentils are low-fat, high in complex carbohydrates and fibre, and have a low GI (see pages 52–53).

• Oily fish is high in essential fatty acids and keeps the brain working.

• Wholegrains are slow-releasing for sustained energy.

• Nuts and seeds are great for your heart.

• Fruit and vegetables protect against heart disease and other chronic illnesses. Eat five portions a day.

REDUCE SATURATED FATS

• Reduces your cholesterol level and reduces your risk of heart disease.

• Replace saturated fats with unsaturated fats, but still watch the calorific values.

REDUCE SALT INTAKE

• Too much salt can cause high blood pressure and associated problems.

• Don't add salt to food and read the labels on processed food.

DETOX FOR A DAY

There are different ways to detox your body, but the basic premises are:

• Give your body a break from trying to metabolize all the snacks and food you are eating.

• Allow your liver to get on with the job it has been designed to do and cleanse your body.

• Living off juices can increase the antioxidants in your body.

THINGS TO AVOID

Dehydration Keep your fluid levels up by drinking little and often. Try keeping a bottle of water with you and don't ignore thirst. Act upon it quickly as it is a sign that your body needs more fluids, preferably water. Sometimes headaches can be caused by dehydration. Another symptom is dark-coloured urine – it should be clear and straw-coloured.

Drinking too much water at once This can wash away essential salts and leave you feeling light-headed.

Over-indulgence This can occur either through eating overly rich foods or just eating too much. Remember the last time you over-indulged? How energized did you feel after that meal? Now remember a time when you ate and drank healthily and notice the difference.

A hangover This is brought on by drinking too much alcohol, which causes severe dehydration, an upset in blood-sugar levels, irritation to the stomach and an overload of toxins. Need I say more?

ENERGIZING FOODS AND DRINKS

What do you do when you need a quick fix of energy? Many people reach for instant energy bars and drinks, and there are convincing arguments as to why these are the answer when your physical energy levels are down. Although they can be good for a quick fix, often you are filling yourself with caffeine and sugar – which provides only a temporary high and results in your body needing to catch up later.

MODERATION IS KEY

The important words here are moderation and balance. Having an energy bar now and then is fine, but if you find yourself eating half a dozen a day, you should consider cutting down, and ask yourself about your overall diet and eating habits.

However, nutritionally speaking there are natural food items that can give you a similar fix without the caffeine and sugar.

USE THE GLYCAEMIC INDEX (GI)

Carbohydrates have a different effect within your body depending on their glycaemic index (GI). This is a system to "rank" food to demonstrate the type of effect the carbohydrate has on blood-glucose levels. A low GI score means that there is a small change in the blood-glucose level after eating certain carbohydrates. This is believed to increase longevity, help weight loss and reduce the risk of heart disease, diabetes and high blood-cholesterol levels. These low-GI carbohydrates also help you to feel full for longer. The following list shows you examples of foods in different categories. Note that low-GI foods are not always healthy – crisps and milk chocolate, for example, are high in fat.

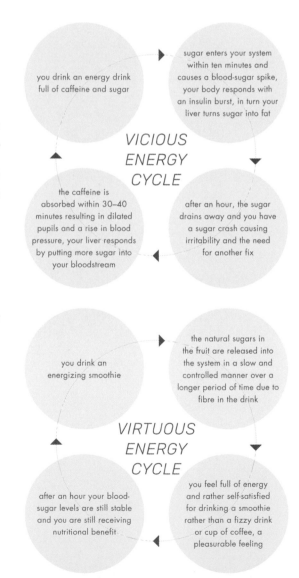

VICIOUS ENERGY CYCLE

you drink an energy drink full of caffeine and sugar

sugar enters your system within ten minutes and causes a blood-sugar spike, your body responds with an insulin burst, in turn your liver turns sugar into fat

after an hour, the sugar drains away and you have a sugar crash causing irritability and the need for another fix

the caffeine is absorbed within 30–40 minutes resulting in dilated pupils and a rise in blood pressure, your liver responds by putting more sugar into your bloodstream

VIRTUOUS ENERGY CYCLE

you drink an energizing smoothie

the natural sugars in the fruit are released into the system in a slow and controlled manner over a longer period of time due to fibre in the drink

you feel full of energy and rather self-satisfied for drinking a smoothie rather than a fizzy drink or cup of coffee, a pleasurable feeling

after an hour your blood-sugar levels are still stable and you are still receiving nutritional benefit

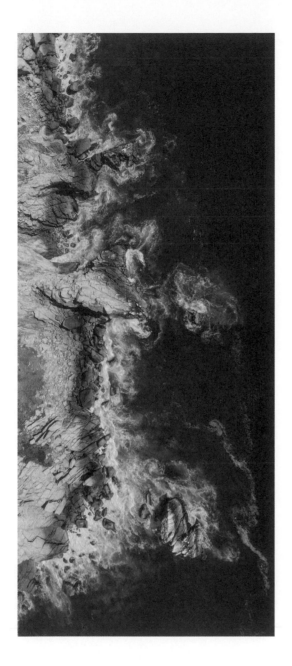

- **Low GI (55 and under) foods include:** low-fat yogurt, dried apricots, soy beverages, potatoes, apples, pears, oranges, spaghetti, sweet potato, basmati rice, lentils, wholegrain bread, baked beans and chickpeas.

- **Medium GI (56–69) foods include:** bananas, melons, pineapples, raisins, new potatoes, oatmeal, popcorn, split peas, brown rice, couscous, wholewheat bread, pitta bread, muesli and honey.

- **High GI (70 and over) foods include:** watermelons, parsnips, swedes, white rice, cereals – bran or cornflakes – white bread, baguettes, white bagels, chips and jellybeans.

EXERCISE TO ENERGIZE

Exercise has many long-term health benefits; it improves body shape, makes you feel good and increases your physical energy level. It can be split up into three types – aerobic exercise, flexibility training and strength training.

TYPES OF EXERCISE

Aerobic exercise increases blood flow to the muscles for extended periods of time and promotes cardiovascular fitness. It needs to be done at regular intervals for at least 30 minutes. The heart becomes stronger and bigger and more effective at pumping blood. Try walking, aerobics, swimming, circuit training, cycling, running or spinning classes.

Flexibility training is about stretching muscles, reducing muscle tension, improving balance, posture and breathing. It improves muscle elasticity, thereby increasing the range of movement and agility. It has a secondary effect of relaxing the mind and the body. Try Pilates, yoga, Tai Chi or Qigong.

Strength training is about increasing the physical strength of muscles. It protects against osteoporosis by increasing bone density, increases muscle size, improves performance, tones appearance and increases muscle support around joints. Use free weights or variable resistance machines.

CORE MUSCLES

The basis for all arm and leg movements is in the centre of the body. Therefore, having a strong core is crucial to good posture, improved sporting technique and avoidance of injury. The muscles deep in your trunk provide this stability and a core stability exercise programme should be included within any exercise programme.

EXERCISE GUIDELINES

Before launching into an exercise programme it is important to reflect on how much training you do already or have done in the past, understand what your objectives are and figure out a way of making exercise one of your good habits.

- Check with your doctor before starting on a strenuous exercise programme.

- Quality, not quantity, is best when carrying out some exercises.

- Warm up and cool down – preparation and recovery help prevent injury.

- Try the talk test – when you are exercising, make sure you can still hold a conversation.

- Balance exercises are important for older people or people with balance problems.
- Your recovery rate should increase as your fitness levels increase.
- Be comfortable in the clothing you wear.
- Exercise at the right intensity level for you – use a scoring guide of 1 to 10, where 1 is sleepy and 10 is flat out.
- Prepare your mind as well as your muscles.

GET MOTIVATED

Motivation is an internal response; it comes from inside you and is about wanting to do something through choice. However much someone else might try to motivate you, they can only inspire you. You must motivate yourself. Here are some common reasons why people are motivated to exercise. Tick the ones that apply to you and add your own at the bottom.

MOTIVATE YOURSELF

○ Get healthy

○ Tone up

○ Lose weight

○ Be stronger

○ Fit into clothes I've grown out of

○ Run with my friend

○ Play with my children in the park

HOW TO STAY MOTIVATED

- Exercise with a friend and do exercise you both enjoy.
- Make it a habit – choose a time and an activity that suits your lifestyle.
- Enter a race, as it gives you a goal to work towards.
- Keep records – immerse yourself in your progress and make it part of your life.
- Set SMART (specific, measurable, attainable, realistic, timely) goals and reward yourself.
- Get the right kit for the exercise – go to a specialist shop if necessary.
- Ask for support from friends and family and get them to tell you how well you are doing.
- Use visualization techniques to help you see the successful and fit you.
- Listen to music – set your personal music player for the right length of exercise time.
- If you get bored, exercise in front of the television for half an hour every night.
- Stay hydrated, but don't over-hydrate yourself and if the exercise hurts, stop – listen to your body.
- If you miss a training session, just let it go and go on to the next.
- Start now! If you are not going to, write down all the reasons why not. Then look at those reasons and turn each one around to make a positive statement about why you are going to do something now. Use the motivation list to help you.

INSTANT ENERGIZERS

There are some things we can do to perk ourselves up quickly. These include exercises to improve breathing, maximizing our oxygen intake, and posture, as well as stretching, which will increase our flexibility before we undertake any more vigorous exercise.

BREATHING

Most of us breathe in a lazy manner and, when you consider how important the breath is, it is very surprising that we are not taught how to breathe properly when we are young. Our breath supplies oxygen to our lungs so that it can be passed around the bloodstream and removes the waste product carbon dioxide. We cannot live without this process. The benefits of breathing well include lowering blood pressure, improving digestion and reducing the effects of stress.

We tend to breathe using the upper part of our lungs rather than the whole of them, which means we are not maximizing our oxygen intake and toxin removal. Ideally, we should take deep, long breaths in through the nose, where the air is filtered and warmed before being transported to the lungs. Then breathe out through the nose.

BREATHING EXERCISES

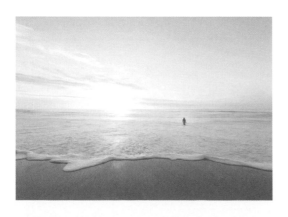

EXERCISE 1

1 Lie flat on your back somewhere comfortable, placing a pillow under your neck for support if you feel any strain.

2 Place your hands below your ribcage on either side of your stomach with your first and second fingertips touching.

3 Take a slow, deep breath in through your nose. You should feel your fingertips begin to separate. If you don't, then you may not be using the full capacity of your lungs. Take another breath and this time make it deeper, while keeping it under control.

4 Lie and breathe in this way for 5 minutes.

POSTURE

Stop, don't move for a moment, and just make a note of your posture. If you are sitting down, is your back straight or are you slumped over this book? A common slumping position is one of a curved back and protruding head, and I am sure most of us have sat like that. So, sit or stand up straight for a moment and feel the difference. Not only will changing your posture reduce the strain you put on parts of your body, but it will also make you look taller and slimmer and feel less tired. Maintain awareness of your posture and keep practising how you stand. Stand in front of a mirror to check your alignment and use shop windows to see how you look when you are walking.

STRETCHING

A good stretch can leave you feeling instantly rejuvenated and full of energy. Easing muscular stresses, improving posture, pumping blood around your body, filling your lungs with air – I can already feel the energy generating while reading about it!

It is fine to carry out stretching exercises if you are healthy and don't suffer from back pain. If you have any concerns in either of these areas, please see your doctor first, especially as joint flexibility can reduce with age. However, taking time out to stretch on a daily basis, as well as making sure you have a good warm-up before, and 5–10 minutes' stretching after, any exercise, will improve your flexibility and limit the effects of age.

Try to stretch every day and hold the stretch so that it lengthens the muscle. Don't bounce to increase the stretch, but wait until the feeling of tension decreases and then increase the stretch a little bit more. Hold each stretch for 20 seconds on each side of the body – if you notice that one side of your body is less flexible, then focus more

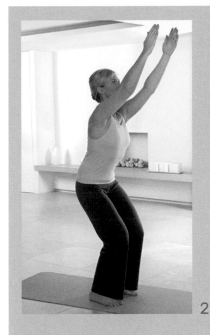

2

EXERCISE 2

1 Stand upright with your feet shoulder-width apart and your arms falling either side of your body.

2 Take a deep breath in while you dip your knees and bring your arms up above your head as you straighten your legs.

3 Release your breath in a smooth, controlled manner as you bring your arms back down to the sides of your body.

4 Do this 10 times, focusing on the depth and quality of the breath.

on stretching that side until you bring your body back into balance. There should not be any pain, just a sense of tension and associated release of tension as you stretch and relax.

STRETCHING EXERCISES

EXERCISE 1

1 Stand tall with your feet together, bend your knees as much as you can without taking your heels off the floor. Feel your stomach muscles pushing back towards your spine and your spine growing longer – take care not to arch it. Do this 8 times.

2 Next, turn your feet out in a V-shape. Make sure to keep your knees over your feet at all times – don't allow them to roll in as this could damage them. Bend your knees, feeling your thigh muscles turn out and your buttock muscles pull under. Bend 3 times, keeping your heels on the floor.

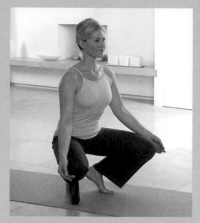

3

3 On the fourth bend, allow your heels to rise and go down as far as you can, keeping your back straight – you may want to hold onto a support to do this. Repeat the sequence twice more.

4 Finally, with your feet about 45 cm (18 inches) apart, turn your legs out from the hip sockets so your knees are over your feet. Bend in the same way as the previous pliés, keeping your heels firmly on the ground, with your thigh muscles turning out. Do not lift your heels at all. Do 4 slow pliés.

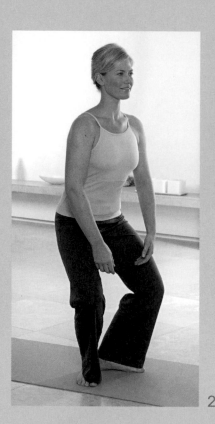

2

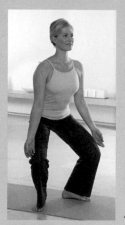

4

EXERCISE 2

1 Stand with your legs hip-width apart
and hold onto the back of a chair or a
table with your fingertips just able to
reach it.

2 Lengthen your spine as far as you can,
with your head dropped to release
any tensions in the neck or shoulders.
Hold the stretch for at least 1 minute,
breathing deeply, and you will feel the
spine extend further.

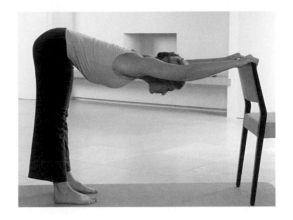

EXERCISE 3

This stretch should not be attempted if you
have any weakness in the back.

1 Position yourself on all fours, knees in
line with your hips, arms in line with
your shoulders, fingers facing forwards.
Your head should be in one long line
from your spine and your spine should
be absolutely straight.

2 Breathing out, pull in your stomach
and form as high and open an arch
with your back as you can.

3 Breathe in as you return to the starting
position then, as you breathe out,
drop your back and lift your head so
that you are looking up. Repeat the
sequence slowly 4 times. If you have
any concerns about the strength of
your back, miss out the second part of
this stretching exercise.

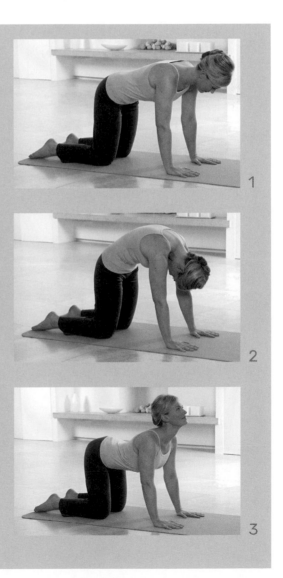

EMOTIONAL TECHNIQUES

This section focuses on how to increase your positive emotional energy and how to preserve that energy by using it wisely. Our emotional state has a direct bearing on our energy levels and the way those levels are channelled. All of us have a finite amount of emotional energy – a resource we need to replenish as much as we can – and use it for positive ends. It is possible to experience many wonderful positive emotions, such as happiness and love, but each positive emotion has its opposite and many of us spend time focusing on negative emotions such as fear and anger.

ANALYSING EMOTIONS

Emotions affect us every day. Take a moment to remember and note down in the box below when you last felt any of the following emotions, where you were, what you were doing and who you were with:

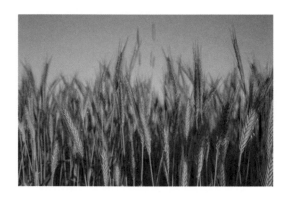

EXAMINE YOUR EMOTIONS

EMOTION	WHERE/WHAT/WHO	EMOTION	WHERE/WHAT/WHO
Amusement		Anxiety	
Awe		Anger	
Desire		Embarrassment	
Excitement		Guilt	
Gratitude		Fear	
Happiness		Hate	
Hope		Irritation	
Love		Loneliness	
Pride		Sadness	

Would you rather have behaved differently than you did? Could you have behaved differently? How did the emotion affect your behaviour and for how long?

Think about an issue you may have had at school or a long time ago and remember the amount of time and energy you expended on it. Consider how important it is to you now and how you could have channelled your energy differently. Was it worth all the upset? Do you feel comfortable with your present ability to recognize your emotions and their effect, and to control your emotions?

Often the heart receives a message before the brain starts to process that message in a logical manner. Recognizing and dealing with these messages is key to managing your emotional energy. There are four main emotions worth exploring in more detail: love, hate, fear and anger. Each affects energy and while each in turn has an energizing element about them, there is also the tendency for destructive or all-consuming emotions.

LOVE

Love is a powerful emotion. It encompasses a feeling of attachment to something or someone, as well as intense passion. Most people spend hours in the pursuit of love. It varies from narcissism to altruism and includes everything in between. Love is amazingly energizing but can have a downside when taken to an obsessive extreme, is unrequited or mixed with jealousy.

HATE

Hate is regarded as the opposite of love, and is a strong aversion to something or someone, or sometimes our hate is born of something we fear. There is a fine line between love and hate – perhaps because, while these emotions are considered opposites, their overwhelming nature is such that they have something in common.

FEAR

Fear is an important emotional response and the key to survival. Our bodies release adrenaline into the blood-stream creating energy to respond to an emergency. All of us experience fear, but it is important to reflect on how appropriate our fears are. For example, being fearful of crossing a busy road where many accidents happen is useful, but fearing a tiny, harmless spider is not.

When you feel fear, you breathe more quickly, so you are able to get oxygen to your muscles, your heart beats faster, which assists in pumping blood more quickly around your body, and your digestive system closes down, allowing you to concentrate on the threat. This is a normal reaction when you are under serious threat. At this point the "fight or flight" reflex comes into play.

ANGER

Anger is another strong emotion and can be passive and aggressive. It has its own function, as it is part of our emotional defences and a way of telling ourselves that we are getting into a physically or emotionally unsafe area. However, when anger controls us and we react without thinking, it affects our life. Learning to resolve conflicts and control our reactions is critical to maintaining high emotional energy levels.

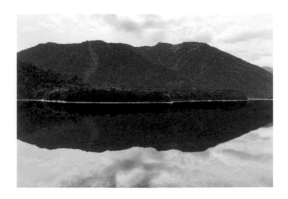

STIMULATE POSITIVE ENERGY

Once you have an understanding of the four main emotions, and how they affect you, you can start to control your emotions rather than allow them to control you. The best way to do this is by maximizing your potential for positive emotional energy. This table provides you with strategies to do this, explains why they work and gives some words of warning.

EMOTIONAL FREEDOM THERAPY (EFT)

This technique was discovered in the 1990s by Gary Craig. It is based on a similar principle to acupuncture, but without needles, and rebalances the body's energy system. It works by tapping on the "energy meridian points" while reliving the negative emotion you want to remove. It can improve some physical and emotional issues, too. For example, it works to help resolve personal problems, reduce stress and restore balance. (A free EFT manual is available online from Gary Craig's website: www.emofree.com.)

AVOIDANCE

While avoidance is not always the answer, sometimes doing something completely different is a good idea. If you are feeling distressed about an issue, it may be worth letting the emotion go and giving yourself space to recover and deal with the issues over time. Rather than ruminating over an upsetting issue, why not go and see a good film?

ASSERTIVENESS

When someone acts in an aggressive way towards us, we often respond in kind. There are also occasions when aggression is met with passivity, or more likely passive-aggressive behaviour; in this case, although someone appears passive on the surface, it is not true underneath. Instead of engaging in this behaviour, work on being assertive.

Keep calm, make assertive statements (see below) clearly and positively and be prepared to repeat if necessary. You should not allow yourself to be brought back into the aggressive/passive-aggressive top of the horseshoe; remain at the base. It will take practice, but it is worth learning this incredibly powerful technique.

- "When you ..." [state the issue]

- "It makes me feel ..." [state your feelings]

- "I would rather you ..." [state what you want and what the positive result would be]

ANGER MANAGEMENT

If you are someone who gets angry and loses control easily, you should consider taking anger-management classes to learn more acceptable forms of behaviour. It will have a major impact on your energy levels.

It may also help you to recognize key triggers that cause you anger, or perhaps situations that cause your stress levels to rise. Try and plan time to deal with these situations and set yourself rules regarding time out when anger energy levels rise.

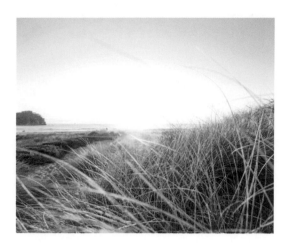

HOW TO MAXIMIZE POTENTIAL ENERGY

STRATEGY	WHY?	HOWEVER...
Accept and take responsibility for your emotional self using terms such as "I feel" instead of "You make me feel".	Taking responsibility for your feelings empowers you to work on them.	Make sure that you are not just over-riding emotions. A bad feeling may be a signal of an intolerable situation that is not good for you.
Show understanding of and empathy with other people.	Only if people are understood will they feel able to express themselves.	Take care not to project your emotions onto others. Remember you are not a therapist; you are there to listen.
Listen to others in a compassionate and non-judgemental way.	People deserve respect for their experiences and views.	Be careful that you don't find yourself in a position of nodding in agreement and inadvertently condoning something that is actually profoundly unacceptable.
Avoid people who bully or railroad you.	This absorbs your emotional energy, and why choose to be a victim?	Sometimes it's a good idea to talk to somebody you trust about your feelings because it may be that you are responding to your own fears.
Pay attention to your feelings when making key decisions.	Your feelings are important – pay attention to all of them.	Paying attention to feelings demands maturity and objectivity.
If you feel out of emotional control be aware that things may have been too much for you.	You deserve self-respect.	Don't try to solve everything yourself – sometimes it is worth stopping and listening to others. You may need to seek help or change the situation.

FEEL-GOOD FACTORS

In our high-pressure world it is often tempting to find short cuts to feeling good and to rest and relaxation, but it is possible to find healthy ways to relax. You can foster good habits for a healthy, productive, constructive, energy-giving future that meet all your needs for social relaxation and long-term sustainability.

ALCOHOL AND STIMULANTS

Many of us fall into the trap of drinking to help us relax. Socializing can often involve spending time with people who are drinking and smoking or even taking illicit substances. The problem is that, over a sustained period, you can come to rely on these quick fixes. You can even become addicted to them, and habits are formed that are not healthy or sustainable over the long term. Such habits sap rather than give energy.

Some patterns of drinking are part of social life. Drinking habits that result from loneliness and isolation or from being part of a strong drinking culture may need special attention – and if you find it hard to stop drinking you may need support.

It is important to recognize and break associations. For example, drinking often goes with smoking, drinking goes with trying to wind down, etc. It may be easier to break the negative habit if you remove yourself from the situation.

ENDORPHINS

The body produces natural painkillers in the brain called endorphins, that work in a similar way to morphine. There are many ways of stimulating an endorphin release in a natural way. For example, by eating chilli peppers; they cause a pain response, which results in an endorphin release. Also, by eating dark chocolate, with a high percentage of cocoa solids, the sugar causes an endorphin release (along with serotonin). The higher the cocoa content the better, as it is full of antioxidants.

Exposing yourself to natural daylight allows sunlight to increase endorphin release and has excellent properties such as converting cholesterol into Vitamin D and enhancing the immune system. Massage can provide a feeling of deep relaxation as well as pain relief and it helps remove toxins. Laughing can also help to reduce stress hormones and can lower blood pressure and boost the immune system.

When exercising, the body is put under stress and then subsequently releases endorphins in response to the pain, resulting in a mood change. Using a transcutaneous electrical nerve stimulator (TENS) machine can also stimulate the body to release endorphins by delivering small electrical pulses.

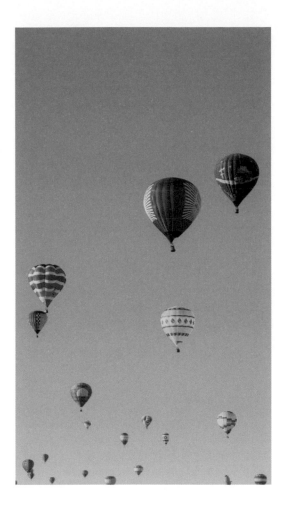

SEROTONIN

Serotonin is a hormone that enhances mood, makes you feel full from food and encourages sleep and relaxation. However, the effect from eating food that releases serotonin varies across individuals. A carbohydrate-rich meal can result in either feeling good or sometimes feeling sleepy. Drinking milk and eating bananas both trigger high releases of serotonin.

GOOD HABITS

Good habits take time to form and you will need to focus on making your habits stick, at least for the first couple of weeks. Try sticking notes around the house with key positive messages.

QUICK WAYS TO FEEL GOOD

There are alternative ways to make you feel good through energizing yourself physically, mentally or spiritually. Here is a selection for you to choose from, or add your own to the list.

- Take a shower, put clean sheets on the bed and open the windows wide.

- Buy a bunch of flowers with a beautiful scent; they will lift your spirits.

- Light a candle; it will lift the energy of a room or burn essential oils, such as ginger. Try bathing by candlelight.

- Incorporate feng shui into your life and live in harmony with your environment by channelling positive energy.

- Have a picnic; sit on the grass or the sand to rejuvenate yourself through direct contact with the energies of the earth.

- Spend time outdoors, go for a walk or go for a swim in the sea.

- Stare at the night sky on a clear night; it is awe-inspiring.

- Sing your favourite song, very loud!

- Spend some time with your favourite person or people.

- Pursue your hobbies, such as reading a good book, or take one up if you don't have one.

- Try reflexology – massaging different points can clear energy blockages.

- Be creative – you will find tips on how to do this in the creative energy techniques section on pages 84–95.

- Take up dancing.

- Give or receive a massage.

REST AND RELAXATION

Your brain needs sleep to remember, concentrate and solve problems. Your body needs sleep to mend injuries, fight sickness and grow muscles, bones and skin. You can see from this that, if your goal is to increase your energy levels, getting sufficient sleep is the most important step you can take.

GETTING ENOUGH?

It is not always easy for us to get enough sleep. We may have small children, or work shift patterns, or have a myriad other reasons that result in insufficient sleep. If this applies to you, you may find your energy levels are seriously affected. One of the first steps in obtaining sufficient sleep is to understand the basic sleep pattern.

GET A GOOD NIGHT'S SLEEP

To be well rested, you should plan your rest time and implement a rest plan that works for you.

- Avoid sugar, alcohol, smoking, caffeine and foods you know will disturb you before bed.

- Sleep in the dark – light prevents melatonin from being produced.

- Don't watch TV before bed – especially stimulating programmes.

- Take a hot bath. This raises the body temperature, which then falls, aiding sleep.

- Go to bed early and get up early. This simulates natural sleeping patterns.

- Keep a routine – go to bed and get up at the same time every day.

SLEEP CYCLES

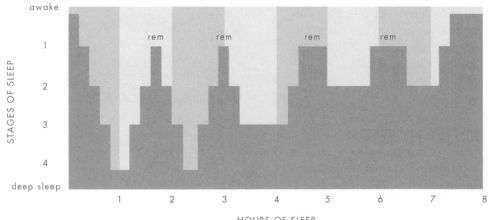

Each cycle is repeated a number of times during the night.

- Maintain a good temperature – ensure the room is at an optimum temperature of 18°C.

- Make sure your bedding is comfortable and your pillows and mattress suit you.

- Make your bedroom a haven of peace and calm – use relaxation music to soothe you.

- Have a notebook and pen beside the bed or some "worry dolls" to share your anxieties.

- Take a glass of water to bed but just sip it to quench your thirst.

- If you wake up in the night don't look at the clock or start clock-watching.

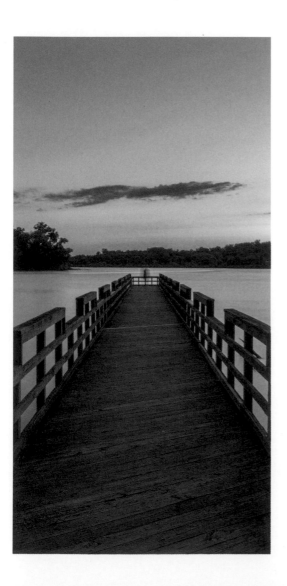

BRING PEACE TO YOUR BODY AND MIND

1. Make yourself warm and comfortable, either lying down on a bed or sitting on a chair.

2. Tense all of your muscles, beginning at your toes and moving up to your face. Keep all your muscles tense. Screw your face up.

3. Relax everything. Take a deep breath in through your nose and out through your mouth. Do this 3 times.

4. Feel each toe relaxing one by one. Move up to your feet and ankles.

5. Feel the tension easing from your muscles as you move up to your calves and then thighs.

6. Continue working your way up your body, focusing on each distinct part in turn. Keep your breathing deep and relaxed.

7. Feel the warmth of your limbs and the relaxation in your body.

8. Remain there for 15 minutes. Acknowledge your thoughts but don't allow them to stay; instead see them drift away.

9. When you feel ready, take 3 deep breaths and feel the energy pass through your body before you gently and carefully rise.

If you are so tense that you don't feel that you can relax and your mind is charged with things that need doing, then you may not feel able to give yourself time to relax. Trying to relax will help the stresses, so try sitting in silence, unmoving, for initially 1 minute a day and then 5 minutes. It is short and simple, but you will be astounded at the results.

BEAT THE "BLUES"

Life is full of highs and lows and it is normal to experience anticlimax or disappointment as well as joy and excitement. It is when the balance of these emotions and experiences is out of kilter that you should think about putting strategies in place to assist you in feeling a little better. Unfortunately, it is often when you are feeling low and most need to change your mood that you feel least able or sufficiently energized to do so.

FEELING LOW?

Everyone feels down sometimes, but the ability to cope with such feelings can depend on your capacity to deal with the low points combined with other issues such as genetic factors, physical, emotional and chemical imbalances, how many events you feel are going against you, illness, stress and fatigue.

DEPRESSION

Depression is a clinical diagnosis and is caused by an imbalance of the brain's chemicals. If you feel that you are suffering from depression it is important to seek medical advice. Symptoms of depression can include:

• loss of energy or feeling lethargic;

• lack of interest;

• change in appetite and sleeping patterns;

• inability to concentrate or make decisions;

• thoughts of suicide.

If you are experiencing several of these symptoms, it is important to go and discuss them with your doctor. There are medical solutions such as antidepressants, which work by balancing the neurotransmitters in the brain, as well as a combination of alternative medicines and therapies such as interpersonal, cognitive behaviour and group therapy.

MOOD SWINGS

Everyone suffers from mood swings from time to time. Often after an enjoyable experience you can find yourself feeling low for no reason. Mood swings can be exacerbated during hormonal changes such as a period, pregnancy or the menopause. If you suffer from mood swings, you will notice changes in your energy level, concentration, anxiety levels and sleep patterns. You may find your self-esteem increases or decreases to a marked extent.

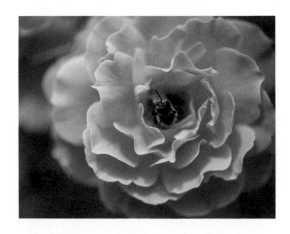

Practical solutions that may help you cope with mood swings could be ensuring you have a good diet, regular exercise and a good night's sleep. You may find that yoga helps you keep your balance in both body and mind.

Try keeping a log of how you feel so that you are able to identify patterns. Increased awareness of how you are affected by mood swings may enable you to manage your changing mood more effectively and interpret how you are feeling differently. If you find your mood swings are severe, you may need to get help from professional sources.

When your mood is low, try to do something to change it. Suggestions include:

• shifting your thought patterns;

• phoning a friend;

• writing a poem;

• doing something that makes you feel good.

YOGA EXERCISE

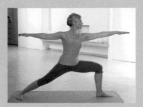

1 Adopt the Warrior pose. Stand with your legs about 1.2 m (4 feet) apart with toes pointing forward. Stretch your arms out sideways in line with your shoulders. Turn your left knee and foot out and bend your knee, keeping your spine straight. Make sure there is a 90-degree angle between your thigh and the floor.

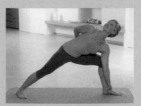

2 Place your left hand on your left ankle, then turn your upper body so you are looking over your right shoulder. You can place your right hand in your inner right thigh to increase the twist. Breathe deeply and hold for 8 seconds.

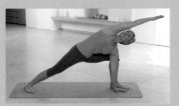

3 Place your left hand on the floor by your foot and extend your right arm by your ear. Look upwards, hold and breathe deeply for 8 seconds.

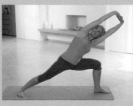

4 Breathe in and raise your body, keeping your spine in the same position. Clasp your hands together and stretch, breathe deeply and hold for 8 seconds. Repeat for the other side.

DEALING WITH STRESS

We often meet stressful situations in life. Our ability to cope with stress is dependent on both our emotional state and our threshold for coping with stress. Whether we have had a good night's sleep and a proper meal affects our ability to deal with stressful situations, as does our environment and the cause of the stress itself.

OVERCOMING STRESS

Identify situations that make you feel stressed. Stop and write down what it is about these situations that stresses you, perhaps using the model on the next page to help you with your problem-solving. Incorporate some relaxation and de-stressing time into your daily routine through some or all of the following.

- Learn relaxation techniques (try the meditation on page 114).

- Eat well.

- Spend time with friends and family (assuming that does not add to your stress!).

- Do things you enjoy.

- Have "feel-good" time (watch a comedy; go to a museum; see an art exhibition).

- Do a puzzle such as Sudoku or crossword to burn off excess mental energy and change your focus.

- Schedule a time for yoga each day.

- Start or rediscover a hobby.

- Listen to your favourite music.

- Practise deep breathing.

- Read a book that grips you.

- Write a card or send an e-mail to someone you haven't seen in a while.

- Clear out a cupboard.

- Plan your next holiday.

HOW DO YOU RECOGNIZE WHEN YOU ARE STRESSED?

FEELINGS	THOUGHTS	BEHAVIOUR	PHYSICAL EXPERIENCE
Out of control	Poor concentration	Irritability	Heart races
Panicky	Fixed on specific worries	Restlessness	Breathlessness
Feeling of doom	Poor attention to others	Not completing key tasks	Tummy upset
Uptight	Thinking something bad may happen	Poor patterns of eating and drinking	Light-headedness
Switched off			General physical unease
Feeling of unreality			

HOW TO RELIEVE A STRESSFUL SITUATION

Here is a technique to help you deal with stressful situations. Once you have completed it, you will find you have clearly laid out a number of options that should help your decision-making process. (Some people find it easier to do this if they pretend they are doing it for someone else.)

1 Identify the situation that is causing you stress and write it in the purple box.

2 Identify four possible solutions to this problem and write each solution in a blue box.

3 Write a list of all the strengths and weaknesses you can identify in each of the proposed solutions in the green and orange boxes, respectively.

4 Consider the four solutions and pick the most suitable one.

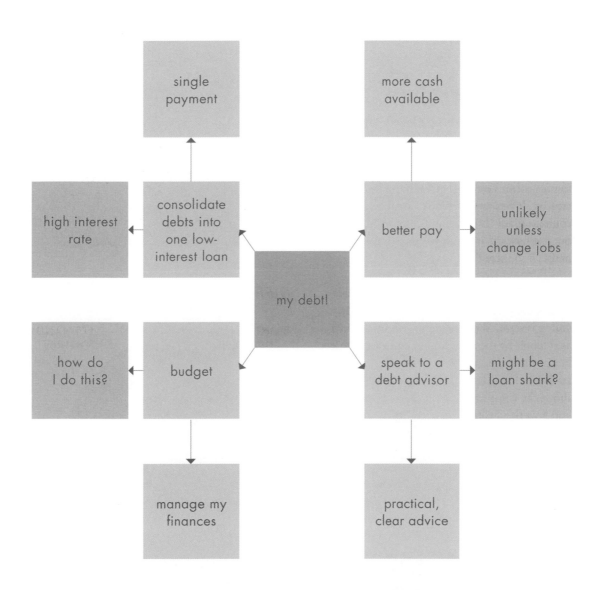

INTELLECTUAL TECHNIQUES

Intellectual energy is not about how high your intelligence quotient (IQ) is, but about having the energy to keep using your brain. Ideally, before embarking on this section of the book, we would take the time to understand how the brain works in detail, but it is incredibly complex. The key point to realize is that the parts of the brain that people use most are the ones that develop. It is thought that older people who play bridge or do newspaper puzzles and have stimulating conversations maintain a high level of functioning for longer than those who don't.

THE HUMAN BRAIN

The brain is an extraordinary organ containing more than 100 billion neurons and weighing approximately 1.5 kg (3 lb). It deals with everything from complex activities and functions to unconscious physical tasks. It can be logical and creative. It was once described as an orchestra – it contains many different and complex instruments, but it is how the instruments work together that makes it so incredible.

For a large percentage of people, the right side of the brain controls the left side of the body, and vice versa. Written language is interpreted as symbols by the right brain and sent to the left brain, while the spoken word is picked up in the auditory channels and sent to the left brain. This shows the complexity of the elements of the brain and how they work together.

Studies have shown that London black-cab drivers have an enhanced part of the brain. The hippocampus, the area responsible for memory, is enlarged owing to their study of what is called "The Knowledge" – the detailed mental road map of the intricate pattern of London streets. The longer they have been driving black cabs around London, the more enlarged their hippocampus is.

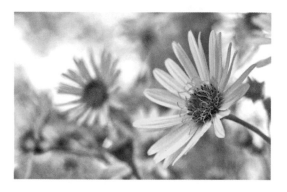

DIFFERENT SIDES OF THE BRAIN

RIGHT-HAND CONTROL

LEFT-HAND CONTROL

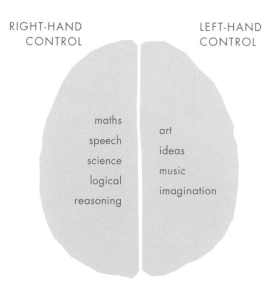

maths
speech
science
logical
reasoning

art
ideas
music
imagination

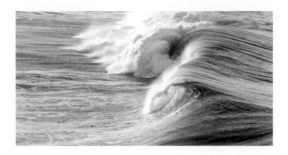

MEMORY

Humans have an amazing memory capacity and, if you consider the quantity of information we take in every day, it is incredible how the brain filters and selects the relevant items to store. It is not always easy to retrieve our memories, although a good trigger is one of our five senses. How many times has hearing a particular song brought back an old memory?

The storage area of the brain is divided into two areas – the short-term and the long-term memories. Initially memories move into the short-term memory and are moved, if relevant or practical enough, to the long-term memory. The short-term or working memory can contain around seven bits of information; this is key to improving your memory – if you can increase what you put in your working memory, then you can remember more for short periods of time.

INTELLIGENCE

Intellectual energy is different from intelligence. However, innate intelligence remains an important part of discussion and understanding of the brain. Expanding the simple view of intelligence, and considering what other experiences form and influence the brain and our intellect, can provide us with a broader and more complex view of intellect. Consider the following points.

• We can measure our intelligence as an underlying IQ value that is set for life.

• We have the ability for multiple intelligences (discovered by Howard Gardner): linguistic (e.g. poet); logical-mathematical (e.g. scientist); musical (e.g. composer); spatial (e.g. sculptor or pilot); bodily-kinesthetic (e.g. athlete); interpersonal (e.g. politician); intrapersonal (to do with oneself); and naturalist (e.g. gardener).

• We can develop intelligence, which depend on the opportunities available to us, our ability to learn, and the people we meet.

• We can transfer skills from one area to another.

• Our intelligence is dependent on that required by our social and cultural norms.

MEMORY STORAGE

STORAGE

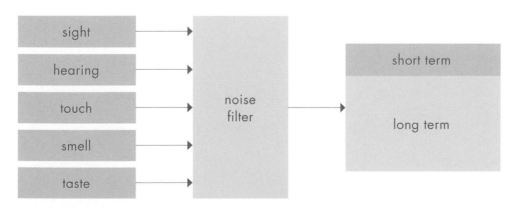

WORK, REST AND PLAY

Concepts of work, rest and play are not as simple as we might think. Some of us enjoy our workplaces and find our home lives stressful and vice versa. It is important to be able to get a balance between those activities that result in an expenditure and net deficit of energy and those that leave you feeling energized. The balance is defined by energy expenditure and gain.

BRING PEACE TO YOUR BODY AND MIND

1 Write down how much time you would like to spend and energy you would like to expend (or gain) in work, rest and play. Use a mark out of 10 for the energy gain or loss. Plot a pie chart for your time and a bar graph for the energy expended and gained.

2 Write down the activities that you have been involved in this week that expended time and energy, and those that generated energy. For example, at work, walking, going out etc. You could keep an activity log for a week and note how much time you spend doing each activity.

3 Categorize them in terms of work, rest and play and plot the time spent, along with how much energy used or gained. This shows where you consider your boundaries are between work, rest and play.

4 Add up the work, rest and play times and draw another pie chart. Compare this with the one from Step 1. Do the same for the energy bar chart and compare. Use colours to differentiate the roles and show you how much energy you spend in each activity. Are there activities that you spend a lot of time on that drain your energy? What gives you energy during the day?

ACTIVITIES	WORK	REST	PLAY	ENERGY +/−
Morning at work	4 hours			−5
Exercise at lunchtime			30 minutes	+2
Shopping			2 hours	+5
Evening out		4 hours		+8

YOUR TIME/ ENERGY RATIO

Did you feel energized, relaxed or tired at the end of the day or week that you plotted? If you feel that you have an energy deficit, look at the amount of time you spend relaxing. If you have a great deal of play-time, do you find it tiring? Nights spent clubbing can leave you exhausted, and sometimes work can give you energy. Which is true for you? People have different energy levels and thresholds. There is no right or wrong answer – it is about understanding yourself.

How do you feel now you have seen your energy versus time levels presented this way? What would your ideal balance be? Plot it now on your ideal energy and time continuum. Think about the adjustments you can make in your life to reach an ideal energized state.

Once you have made these changes, revisit the reflection and awareness technique, and see how you have improved.

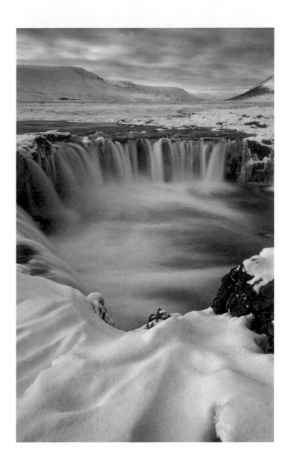

TOP TIPS FOR GETTING THE BALANCE RIGHT

Some countries have a culture of "face-time" meaning that people spend very long hours at work. Yet it is often ineffective to work longer rather than in a more focused and timely manner.

• If possible, do the work you love. When boundaries between work and play blur, energy levels remain high and you are fortunate. (While this is the ideal, many of us are less fortunate, finding our energies sapped by work and needing to focus on recharging our energies by other means.)

• If you work from home, build boundaries between work, rest and play. Close a door, if possible, so that you can "leave" the office.

• Don't procrastinate – so much energy is wasted thinking when sometimes you would have completed the job by just doing it.

• Be efficient – inefficiency costs time, energy and money. Set a schedule and stick to it.

• Be strict with your time – try out the time-management techniques on pages 90–91.

FEED YOUR BRAIN

A good diet is important for both the development and functioning of the brain. Around two-thirds of the brain's material is made up of fatty acids, which are used for communication. There are two essential fatty acids that cannot be made in the body and therefore have to be consumed. The first is alpha-linolenic acid, known as the "omega-3" family of fatty acids. The second is linoleic acid, known as the "omega-6" family of fatty acids.

The brain combines these two groups of fatty acids to build long-chain fatty acids that actually make up the substances of the brain. However, the ability to do this depends on good overall nutrition and a correct proportion of omega-3 and omega-6 fatty acids. Unfortunately, in modern diets we tend to consume a much larger proportion of omega-6 than we need. So, try to increase your consumption of omega-3 and reduce your omega-6 intake. Studies have shown that a deficiency in essential fatty acids (EFAs) is associated with a spectrum of behavioural disorders including attention deficit hyperactivity disorder (ADHD), dyslexia and dyspraxia. We also eat a lot of man-made trans fatty acids (in chips/French fries, margarine and crisps cooked in hydrogenated oil), which can disturb communication in the brain (as well as clogging up the arteries), causing heart disease and making people overweight.

Keep your blood-sugar levels constant by snacking on dried fruit and/or cereal bars, keep your brain hydrated by drinking plenty of water and stimulate your interest in healthy foods by including variety.

VITAMINS AND MINERALS FOR GOOD BRAIN HEALTH

Vitamin B – found in liver, kidneys, vegetables, wholegrains and dairy products.

Vitamin C – found in fruit.

Vitamin E – found in olive oil, corn oil, nuts, seeds and wheatgerm.

Magnesium – occurs in green leafy vegetables, nuts, bread, fish, meat and dairy products.

Zinc – occurs in oysters, red meat, poultry, beans, nuts and wholegrains.

ESSENTIAL FATTY ACIDS

Omega-3

Sardines   Salmon   Mackerel   Herring   Anchovies   Tuna*   Linseed   Walnuts   Soya beans   Leafy greens

Omega-6

Sunflower oil   Corn oil   Soya oil   Evening primrose oil   Wheatgerm

* Pregnant women should note recommended intake limits

PLAN A MEDITERRANEAN DIET DAY

A typical Mediterranean diet includes foods such as fresh fruit, vegetables, fish, nuts, seeds, olive oil, wholegrains and red wine (in moderation). It is full of essential fatty acids and antioxidants, and is good for the heart. Why not try eating the Mediterranean way today?

BREAKFAST

- Natural low-fat yogurt
- Fresh fruit
- Handful of nuts
- Freshly squeezed orange juice

LUNCH

- Salad of tomatoes, feta cheese, fresh basil and extra virgin olive oil dressing
- Pasta with pine nuts, extra virgin olive oil, sun-dried tomatoes, chopped peppers and olives

SNACK

- Hummus with pitta bread and carrot sticks

DINNER

- Fish roasted in lemon juice and mixed herbs with roasted vegetables
- Cherries and plums

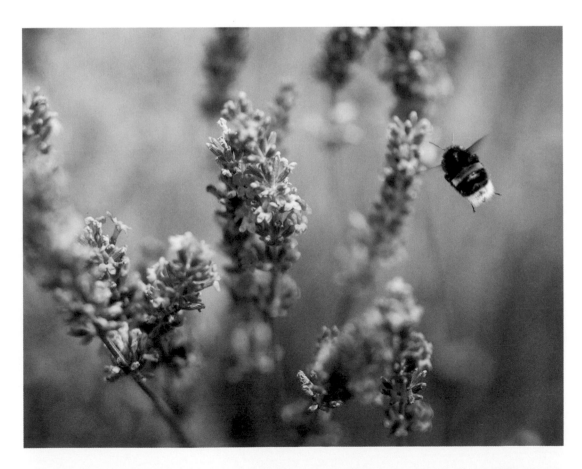

ENERGIZE YOUR SPACE

Being comfortable in our surroundings can aid our intellectual, creative and emotional energies. Wherever we spend our working life, balance and harmony are important in order to think clearly and concentrate. There are ways we can all improve our mental clarity and performance by making small adjustments to the immediate area.

MAKE SPACE

One of the most important things you can do is to clear clutter and be organized. Being tidy means you don't waste time looking for things and also makes you feel in control. Some people are amazed at how much more efficiently they are able to think when they have empty space around them to work in.

Start now! Begin by tidying a small area and finish that before you tackle the next. Recycle whatever you can, but shred sensitive documents. If you feel panicky about letting something go, keep it stored away for six months and see whether you really need it during this time. Next see what you can do about any distractions within your line of sight. Lastly, review your filing and storage arrangements.

ARE YOU SITTING COMFORTABLY?

Aim to make your work area as pleasant as possible while keeping it fit for purpose. In particular, look at ways of avoiding physical strain and maintaining good posture. If you are constantly squirming in discomfort, you will never get anything done.

- Your chair should support your back and your feet should be in complete contact with the floor when your legs are bent at 90 degrees from the knees.

- Check that your desk, computer screen and keyboard are all at the right height and take regular breaks.

- Avoid screen glare by fitting a filter or adjusting window blinds and curtains, and ensure that lighting arrangements are adequate and don't cause eyestrain.

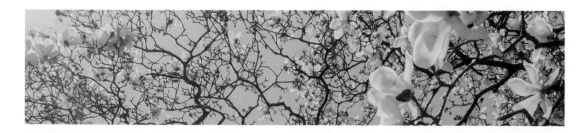

ENERGIZE THE ATMOSPHERE

There is nothing like a breath of fresh air to keep you stimulated and alert, so make sure you are getting enough oxygen. If background noise is a problem, take steps to minimize its impact.

Research carried out by NASA discovered that some houseplants remove certain organic pollutants from the air. This has been shown to help alleviate the "sick building syndrome" that has been associated with many new, poorly ventilated buildings.

Chrysanthemums, bamboo palms (*Chamaedorea* spp.), Chinese evergreen (*Aglaeonema modestum*) and gerberas are particularly effective.

Scientists have found that a lack of negative ions in the bloodstream impairs our ability to deliver oxygen to the cells and tissues, decreases the production of serotonin and reduces our immunity to disease. Employees of organizations that have installed negative air ionizers are less likely to get colds, absent less frequently and are generally more cheerful and alert.

PURIFY THE ATMOSPHERE

Try to keep the area well ventilated – a flow of fresh air will help to remove toxins and ensure the air is not too dry or humid.

Open a window if you can and replace the "old" air with fresh air.

Plants have many energizing properties. They provide colour to lift mood, remove carbon dioxide and produce oxygen to stimulate brain activity.

Keep the air temperature at a comfortable level – too warm or too cold and you will feel sluggish and unable to concentrate.

Consider using an ionizer to charge the air with negative ions and to improve alertness, mood and health.

Even if you don't have much control over your surroundings try adding objects to your desk or pictures to help raise your energy levels.

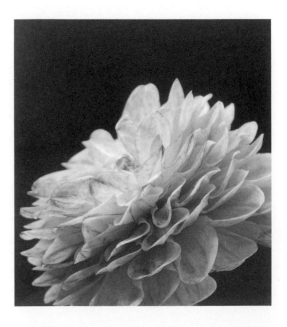

LIFTING LEMON

To feel more alert, try using aromatherapy. Research has shown that lemon activates the centre of the hippocampus (the part of the brain connected with learning and memory). Lemon oil is commonly diffused through air-conditioning systems in Japanese workplaces after scientists discovered that typists made 54 per cent fewer errors when subjected to it. Research also shows that the scent of lemon lowers blood pressure, relaxes the brainwaves and has an antidepressant effect. (For the energizing properties of herbal remedies, see pages 114–115.)

STIMULATE YOUR BRAIN

Whether they are electric, diesel or steam, all trains need fuel to move forward and pull the carriages attached to them. Your brain is the engine – the more work your brain has to do, the more energy it will need. If you imagine your brain is the engine, how fast is your train moving? What fuel are you putting in? If you are struggling to pull the carriages of life at the moment, what are you going to do if there is a hill ahead?

FUEL YOUR BRAIN TRAIN

- Read books to improve language and concentration.

- Exercise to increase oxygen and blood flow to the brain.

- Sleep – a good night's sleep is imperative for proper brain functioning.

- Drink water to keep your brain hydrated.

- Listen to music. We frequently associate things with music and that is why they sometimes come back so quickly.

- Carry out the mental gym exercises on pages 82–83.

THE RABBIT

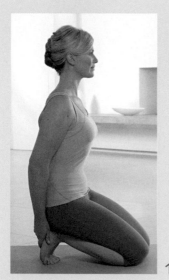

1 Kneel on the floor with your toes tucked underneath. Clasp your hands around your heels and sit up straight.

2 Inhale, then as you exhale curl your spine and place your forehead on the floor. Try and get it as close as possible to your knees. Breathe normally.

3 Carefully roll on to the top of your head, straightening your elbows and raising your hips. Hold for 20 seconds while breathing deeply. Repeat the exercise.

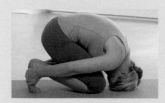

HEADSTAND

1 Kneel on the floor, lace your fingers together with your thumbs crossed and place your arms on the floor.

2 Place your head onto the floor in front of your hands. Make sure that your elbows are directly below your shoulder blades.

3 Tuck your toes under, then come up onto your toes with your legs straight. Then carefully walk your feet towards your head until your spine is straight.

4 Bend your right knee up and then the left. Keep your knees and feet together and raise your legs up together. Drop your feet behind you.

5 Straighten your legs. You should not have your weight resting on your head, your arms should be supporting you.

6 Breathe normally and keep in the position for as long as possible. Then, slowly drop your feet back behind you, bring your knees forward and curve your spine to return to the floor. Don't stand up immediately, as you may feel dizzy.

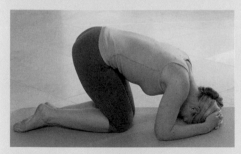

1

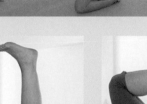

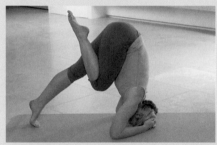

2

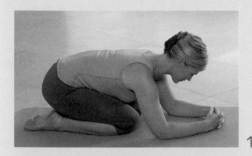

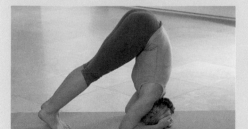

4

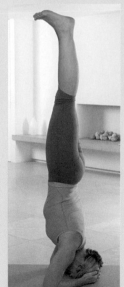

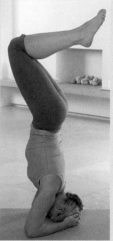

5

6

MENTAL GYM EXERCISES

Here are some techniques to help keep you fit and healthy intellectually.

THE NAME GAME

When you meet someone, repeat their name immediately they tell you it, and then visualize something distinctive about them and make the picture as ridiculous as possible. Try to use their name again during the next couple of minutes and see the picture again to fix their name in your brain.

HANDY REMINDERS

Use stickies to make your notes. They were initially designed in yellow for a good reason – the colour alerts your visual system and helps you remember.

BRAIN EXERCISE

Buy yourself an electronic "play" device that features activities designed to stimulate your brain and give it a workout (such as solving simple maths problems, drawing pictures on the touch screen and reading classic literature out loud).

NOW CONCENTRATE

Set yourself a task and a time to work on, or complete, the task. Focus on just that task and ignore everything else. Perhaps put a timer on so that you don't have to check the clock. When your time is up, treat yourself to a quick walk or a cup of tea as a break.

GET REACTIVE

Get someone to help you. Ask them to hold a glove or ruler at arm's length and drop it. Your aim is to catch it before it hits the floor. Stand further away and repeat, to see if you can improve your reaction time.

LEARNING STYLES

We all have a preferred way of learning, and recognizing this helps us learn things more quickly and simply. Peter Honey and Alan Mumford devised a questionnaire to help people determine their preferred learning style. They describe four different styles:

Activist – likes to be doing things and be involved in new ideas.

Reflector – likes to collect information and think about it carefully.

Theorist – likes to think through problems logically and analytically.

Pragmatist – likes to try things out and get on with things practically.

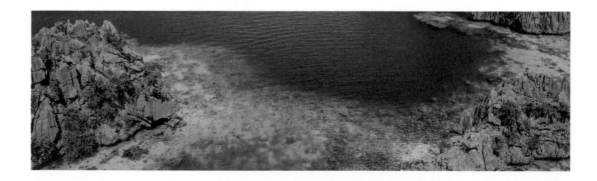

Accelerated learning is a form of learning where all the brain is stimulated, which fires off connections between the two halves of the brain. Rather than just reading from a textbook, practically experiencing something means learning by doing and making it memorable on the way. Try to learn new things in an active way, stimulating as many of the five senses as possible. People have a different ability to learn dependent on an innate preference – visual, auditory, tactile, kinesthetic. Absorb yourself in your learning. Make it enjoyable.

IMPROVE YOUR MEMORY

Improving memory takes practice, but there are many ways of aiding the build-up of memory. Think of it as a muscle that needs exercising and nurturing to build up its strength. Use different senses to stimulate your memory and keep practising. Try the ideas shown below.

MOTOR MEMORY

Try to remember a poem while doing a certain physical exercise. You will find that you will associate each line with a different motor movement.

RECALL LISTS

Group similar items under headings to help recall lists. Try linking items by making up a story. Use mnemonics, such as "Richard Of York Gave Battle In Vain" for the colours of the rainbow (red, orange, yellow, green, blue, indigo, violet).

MEMORY GAMES

- Take a tray and put 10–20 small items on it. Look at the tray for 60 seconds. Cover the tray and write down what you saw.

- Lay out a pack of cards face down. Turn over two cards at a time to try to make a matching pair. Keep going until you have paired all the cards up. (See what effect lying the cards randomly versus putting them in rows has on your memory.)

- With one or more other players, say "When I went shopping I bought ..." and add an item. The next player repeats the sentence, any previous items and adds one. Keep going until you can no longer remember the list. (Use the list trick above of making up a story.)

TOP TIPS FOR IMPROVING YOUR MEMORY

Understand your memory and what you are good at (short-term, long-term, visual, verbal).

- Concentrate at times of the day when you feel your brain functions at its best.

- Rehearse information in your mind by repeating it over and over again.

- Use mnemonics (a memorable short poem or word) to remember lists by associating the information with the poem or word.

- Learn by rote (e.g. times tables).

- Practise learning telephone numbers.

- Declutter and organize, it will have a major impact on your mental capacity.

CREATIVE TECHNIQUES

Creativity is the use of our minds for inspiration, ideas, invention and imagination. It is literacy, painting, performance, gardening, dancing and sculpting. Visit any nursery class and you will find artwork all over the walls and paint all over fingers. At some point most of us feel we stop being creative beings. Yet the houses we live in, the cars we drive in, almost everything we look at and see has been created by the power of the mind. Look around you, almost everything you see is made or has been grown and nurtured by humans. Each of them started as a creative idea or thought in someone's head.

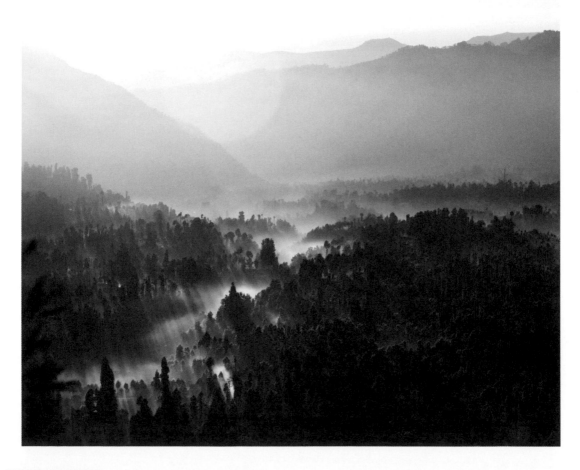

START TO FEEL CREATIVE

If you scored low on creative energy, don't fool yourself into thinking this is how it is. Don't make the mistake of thinking that you are not a creative being. Instead, find your "inner child" and recognize what it is that stops you feeling creative. Spend a moment writing down the reasons why you feel you are not creative.

Now, turn each of those phrases around to say how you could overcome these blockages. If you are struggling to do this, imagine the most creative person you know and write down how they would act. Pretend you are someone else. It feels very different when we start to change our mindset and overcome some of our mental blocks.

CREATIVE ENERGY BENEFITS

It allows you to think "outside the box" – you can look at the world in a different way with a different perspective. It could be the difference between looking at a clock and just seeing the time, and looking at the clock and understanding how the clock works, or thinking of the concept of time and how it affects people.

You may be able to find solutions to problems that appear impossible; the answer might be lurking around a corner if you just think in an alternative way. Your personal and professional life could be taken in a new direction in life that is full of reward and fulfilment, while giving you the opportunity to discover more about yourself.

TOP TIPS FOR IMPROVING YOUR CREATIVE ENERGY

- Make your environment, including noise or music levels, comfortable and stimulating.

- Declutter so you have space for your creative activity.

- Believe in your creative self – look at yourself in the mirror and tell yourself why you are creative, and how you will use your creative energy. Say it out loud and believe it.

- Talk to people – chat generates new ideas and gives you opportunity to bounce those ideas around.

- Persevere – it takes time to learn a creative skill.

- Practise, practise, practise – if you are enjoying yourself, it will not even feel like practising.

- Be satisfied with yourself – don't expect everything to be perfect. I remember being in a pottery class once and we were told to mould a part of our anatomy out of clay, with our eyes closed. I sculpted the most beautiful, elegant foot that had ever been made. When I opened my eyes I was met with a rather ugly, misshapen, foot-like protuberance. I did not keep the pottery, but if I close my eyes I can still see the one in my imagination.

- Learn skills – a lot of creativity is based on acquired skills. There are classes in a huge variety of subjects. Why not go to an art class or whatever other creative task you may be interested in?

- Be inspired! Go to new exhibitions or talk about films with your friends, for example.

- Do something out of the ordinary.

STIMULATE YOUR CREATIVITY

So, you have understood the benefits of increasing your creative energies and read through the top tips. If you still feel a bit "stuck", below you will find some strategies to stimulate creativity within you.

EXERCISES TO GENERATE IDEAS

The following exercises are meant to help you generate creative ideas for any problem or issue you have. Form your problem into a clear statement and write it down on a piece of paper. Then choose one, or more, of the following exercises to help you generate solutions. At this stage they don't have to be meaningful; allow your mind to be creative.

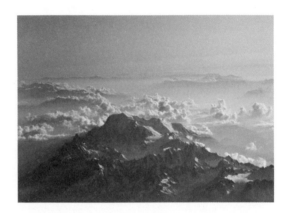

BE CREATIVE

- First thing every morning for two weeks, write anything you can think of on a side of A4. Don't read it, just put it away.

- Recognize the barriers that are stopping you (see "Dealing with blockages" on page 92) and do something to remove them.

- Believe in yourself and use positive attitude and language.

- Use emotion.

- Understand that there are no right or wrong answers; just create.

- Be with people you feel comfortable with.

- Produce the right conditions and environment for you.

- Programme yourself to think creatively (use the visualization techniques on pages 94–95 and 118–119).

- Be aware of the difference between left- and right-brain thinking (see page 72), and use tools to trigger a shift in emphasis.

- Believe that you attract what you think about, so think of yourself as a creative being.

- Visit somewhere inspirational.

- Listen to classical music.

- Go for a walk.

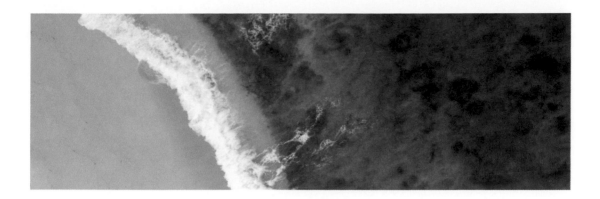

BRAINSTORMING

Brainstorming is about letting your creative mind pour all your ideas out. Don't stop to think about how practical the ideas are, as they can always be removed later.

- Brainstorm as a list.
- Use sticky notes for each idea and stick them on the wall.
- Scatter your ideas over a piece of paper, keeping them random.
- Try brainstorming with other people and bounce ideas off each other.

PLAY-DOH

Take a number of sets of Play-Doh and mould shapes while you think about your problem. Make notes about any thoughts that come to mind. You could even start to shape your answer with the play dough, if possible.

DRAWING

Try drawing your problem and the ideal solution, as described on page 88.

GENIE AND THE LAMP

Think of your problem and give yourself three wishes to solve it. Remember a genie is magical, so don't limit or constrain yourself.

SUPERHERO TECHNIQUE

Write down your problem and then take on the mantle of your favourite superhero. Answer the problem in the manner in which they would. For example, Superman might fly through the air.

ROLE PLAY

Try acting out possible solutions to the problem, making it as real as possible. Ad lib as you go along and speak out loud. Incorporate others in this if possible.

WHY, WHY, WHY?

State your problem and ask "Why?" Write your answer down. Ask, "Why?" Keep repeating this exercise until you run out of time or answers.

Set time aside to take your pile of solutions and look at them one by one, reflecting on any thoughts that are triggered. Choose three or four solutions that are suitable for further consideration and mark them with coloured stickers and stars. These may well be your solutions, ask yourself the following questions.

- Can you implement them?
- When?
- How?

ACHIEVE YOUR GOALS

It is hard to achieve what you want in life unless you take the time to think what your goals are and set them. Goals need to be realistic while still allowing you your dreams. Write your goals down now (start each one with an imperative such as "make" or "decide"), and divide them into manageable chunks to help you focus and reward achievement.

GOALS SHOULD BE SMART

Specific – what are you going to do, and why? How are you going to do it?

Measurable – you need to be able to measure whether you have reached your goal.

Attainable – make your goals feasible; they should stretch you, but not be so out of reach that you feel disillusioned.

Realistic – for example, never eating chocolate again might be less realistic than limiting the chocolate you eat.

Timely – put a timeframe on your goal.

PLAN MORE THAN ONE GOAL

If you have more than one goal, produce a time plan for yourself. In the example below, the first goal is to lose a certain amount of weight, the second is to change or improve jobs and the third is to take up a creative pastime. Using this method, you can see what tasks need to be done to achieve your goals and include interim steps to make it easier to reach your end point.

DRAW YOUR GOAL

Drawing your goal and your path to get there is a creative way of working out the best way to achieve it. This technique works well with life goals and dreams that have more than one element. You don't need great artistic skills – just the ability to draw stick figures. If this is too much, cut out pictures from magazines and make a collage. Draw six boxes, placing a picture of your required outcome in Box 6. Then draw a picture of where you are now in Box 1. Lastly draw pictures in Boxes 2–5 of how you are going to get from Box 1 to Box 6.

JAN	FEB	MAR	APR	MAY	JUN
Lose 2 kg (4 lb) by end of month			Reach goal weight 63.5 kg (10 stone)		
		Research three new job roles by 15 March			

JUL	AUG	SEP	OCT	NOV	DEC
Start new job by 1 July					
		Start creative training class by end of month			

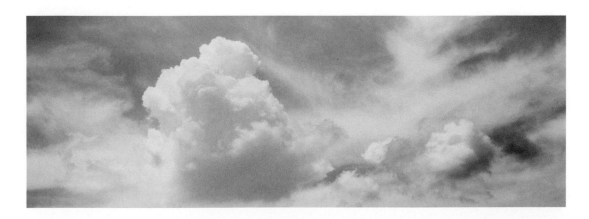

MANAGE YOUR TIME

The most important key to getting things done is time management. The better you can arrange your time, the more time there will be for you to lose yourself in your creative activities.

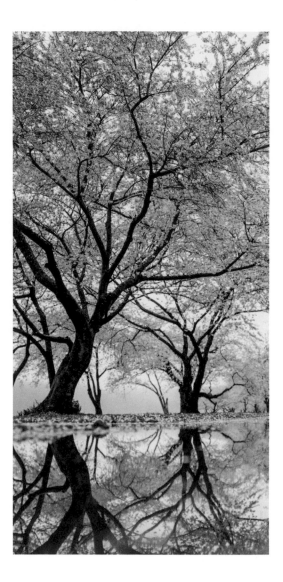

LOG YOUR TIME

Find out how much time you really spend doing things. Start a journal in the morning and make a note of how long you spend on breakfast, travelling, coffee breaks, working at your desk and so on. Do this for a whole week without referring to it and then look back and review your time management. How did you do? Can you see any wasted time or room for efficiencies?

PRIORITIZE

Find a quiet place and list all the things you have outstanding, whether they be urgent issues that need dealing with now or long-lasting dreams that you would like to achieve one day.

TRAFFIC-LIGHT PRIORITY SYSTEM

RED	AMBER	GREEN
Book dentist appointment	Organise birthday party	Visit a local monument
Complete work assignment	Update CV	Learn to sail

Just let your mind flow and capture them all on paper. You can do this by writing them as a list or drawing them. Even if some of them seem quite daunting, record them – you can always break them down into smaller, manageable chunks (see page 88 for more information on achieving goals).

If you prefer, you can be selective about what you put on the main list. There may be some goals that are for longer-term planning, and you may want to capture those on a separate list. It is up to you.

Once you have captured as many as possible (you can add to this at any time), you need to prioritize. When considering how to prioritize, you can either "cherry pick" by taking your list and putting the tasks in the order that you want to carry them out, or you can use the "traffic light" system in which there are three priority levels of red, amber and green, where red is high priority and green is low priority.

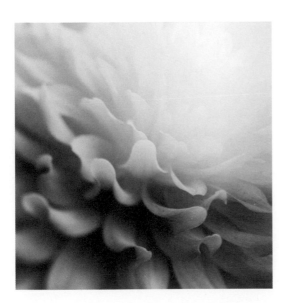

- Do the worst thing first – there is usually one task that you don't want to do more than any other. Every morning, do the thing you are putting off – it is very liberating.

- Plan your time – timetable hours to complete different tasks and try to stick to this.

- Improve your decision-making – write down the pros and cons and make an assessment. If you don't make a decision, you are deciding not to act on a problem or task. If you need support, try using one of the problem-solving techniques on page 87.

- Set deadlines and stick to them.

- Allow time for unforeseen events – there are always interruptions in life.

- Throw away – if you have a tendency to keep things just in case they are useful, give yourself a "just in case" box and keep them in there. Every six months or when the box becomes too full, throw away things that are not useful.

- Learn to say no! Don't take on too much, consider what your priorities are and say no when appropriate.

- Learn not to procrastinate.

- Identify what excuses you make to yourself and find a way to overcome them.

BLAST THOSE BLOCKAGES

We have all experienced that disheartening feeling when a little voice inside our head says, "I can't do it!" Something prevents us from letting go and being freely creative. It takes time, practice and energy to keep creativity alive and to overcome a blockage. Use the outside world to help you – books, the internet and people can be an excellent source of creativity.

FEAR

Often our childhood memories are the main blockage to our creativity. Remember time spent painting, sticking collages together or writing stories? Unfortunately, fear often holds us back from experimenting again. We should be grateful to this fear, however. It is there to protect us and was probably learned from an early experience where we did not feel our creations were good enough. So, next time your fear stops you from trying, stop and think, why not have a go? Thank your fear for protecting you. Recognize that it has been doing a good job and let it go. This may take some practice but each time it will get easier.

WRITER'S BLOCK

This is a where a writer sits with a blank page or screen in front of them, feeling the pressure to perform, without any free creative flow. The trick is just to start – write anything down. It is much easier to edit something than sit looking at a blank piece of paper or screen.

EXTERNAL FACTORS

Blockages don't just come from within; they can also stem from our environment, from being part of an organization, from a social setting or even from other people. It takes time, practice and energy to keep creativity alive and overcome that fear.

FINISH WHAT YOU START

The final thing that can block us is our ability to close down on our creativity. It is good to generate lots of ideas, but the down side can be a lack of focus and decision-making. Remember, completing and finishing tasks is just as important a part of creativity.

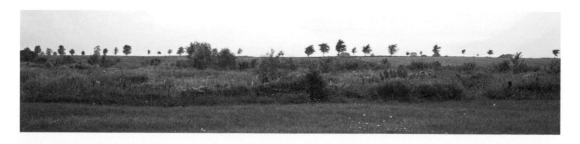

TOP TIPS FOR DEALING WITH BLOCKAGES

- Do some deep breathing exercises (see page 56) or meditate.

- Separate yourself from whatever it is that is blocking you for a while.

- Draw or write with your "wrong" hand.

- Put on an inspiring piece of music or just daydream.

- Yell out loud.

- Go for a walk or go swimming.

- Ask someone to come and help you.

- Use past experiences to help you.

- Keep a scrapbook and record anything interesting you see, hear or read.

YOGA EXERCISE

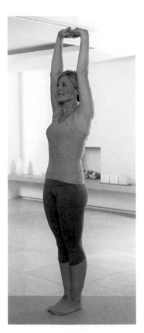
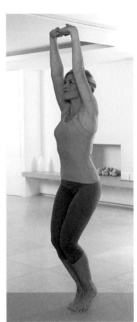
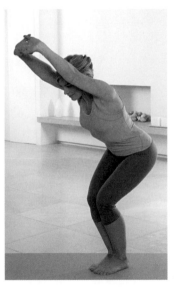

1   2   3

1 Stand up straight, stretch your arms above your head and clasp your fingers together. Keep your shoulder blades down and your elbows straight and close to your ears. Hold for 5 seconds.

2 Inhale, then rise up onto your toes while breathing deeply. Hold for 5 seconds. Then, lift your heels a little higher and bend your knees.

3 Drop your heels back down and stretch your hips backwards, increasing the depth of your breathing. Make sure your spine stays straight and your arms stay in line with your ears. Hold for 20 seconds. Repeat the exercise.

VISUALIZATION EXERCISES

Spend a moment vividly imagining the creative you. Make it as real as you can. How do you look? What are you wearing? How do you feel? You have just carried out a visualization exercise, and it was probably a lot easier than you thought it would be. It is a way of connecting your thoughts, dreams, desires and emotions – all you need next is the action. Even that is not difficult since, by starting to visualize your dreams, you have already begun to change your pattern of behaviour. Once you can visualize something, then it can manifest itself.

MORNING RITUAL

Decide that you are going to set yourself a morning ritual. This is going to benefit you in two ways. It will help you with your creative visualizations and it will give you an energy burst every morning. Ask yourself the following questions.

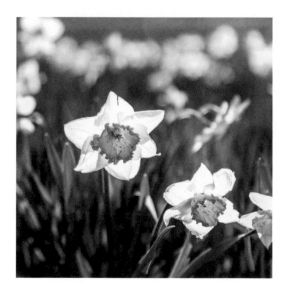

- How do I want to feel when I wake up in the morning?

- What would be my favourite way to wake up?

- What will I do when I get out of bed?

- How great am I going to feel?

- What am I going to eat that is healthy for breakfast?

- What exercise am I going to do?

Spend some time focusing on your ideal morning (which should not be one of lying in bed with a hangover); remember this is the first step to changing your behaviour patterns.

Some ideas that you could include in your morning ritual include: exfoliating the skin with a loofah; using a body brush or salt body scrub; covering yourself in Moor mud (said to nourish and rejuvenate tissues, detox and reduce inflammation); or alternating your shower between hot and cold to invigorate your body and mind.

Now tell yourself, out loud, that you are going to start your morning ritual tomorrow morning... and make it happen.

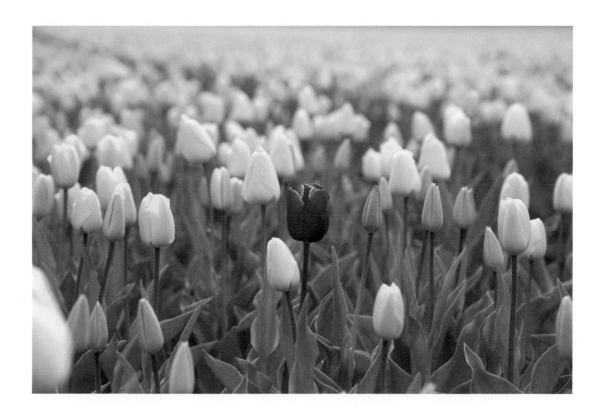

MAKE A DREAM BOARD

A dream board is a creative visualization of your hopes and aspirations. It is a powerful way of tapping into the depths of your mind by covering a large board in pictorial images of your dreams and goals. Be creative in your visualizations and use props to help you make something visually pleasing, like a dream board.

1 Buy a cork board and some pins as a basis for your dream board.

2 Visualize your dream and search for photos, articles, colours – anything that symbolizes your dream – to put on your board.

3 Make it as specific or as general as you want.

4 Add a timeline so you know when you want to achieve your dream or dreams.

5 Make sure you include all the aspects of your life; make it a balanced dream.

6 Make your dream board so that you love to look at it and you feel the emotions that have made it. Have fun making it.

7 Put your dream board where you are going to see it every day, especially in the morning so that you can feel good about the day and your future; and in the evening so it is the last thing you think about at night.

PERSONAL TECHNIQUES

Your personal energy profile is based on you, living as your authentic self. What does this mean? Well, do you live by your values and beliefs? Do you spend time doing what you really love doing? What is it that makes your heart sing? How much time do you spend in positive encounters? Understanding self and taking time out for you is an important step in freeing your personal energy. Now is the time to fuel your success and realize your potential.

THINK POSITIVE

What positive words can you think of that link to self? Here are a few possibilities: self-esteem, self-respect, self-discipline, self-confidence, self-worth, self-determination.

How do these words make you feel? Spend a moment on each in turn, judging yourself on the extent to which you consider you have that quality. Be honest with yourself and identify gaps where you consider there is room to develop further.

Our sense of self influences the way we approach life, set goals and search for increased understanding of our purpose. As we grow older, and we hope wiser, our experiences and insights continue to have bearing on what we truly want from life and on the extent to which we accept that and work towards it.

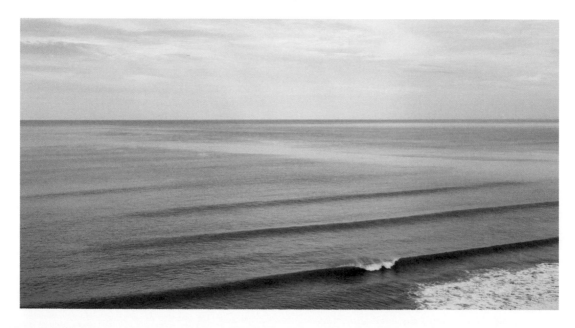

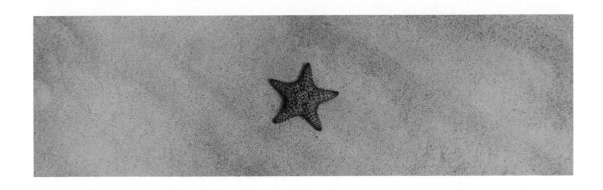

HOW TO IMPROVE YOUR PERSONAL ENERGY

- Be happy with who you are – don't compare yourself with others, but accept yourself for yourself.

- Surround yourself with people who make you feel good about yourself, who make you feel successful and loved.

- Go out of your way to make other people feel good about themselves.

- Ignore your critical voice – we all have a voice inside our heads that puts us down. Switch this voice off or turn the volume down. Imagine that you have a radio tuner in your head and, when the voice is not being helpful and positive, change channels.

- List your strengths, and ask five people to tell you what they believe your strengths are. (If they volunteer your weaknesses, then, as every strength is also a weakness, so every weakness is also a strength. Consider how any weakness identified may sometimes be a strength.) Keep the lists to read at regular intervals and remind yourself of your uniqueness.

- Search out energy angels (see page 106) when you are feeling low.

- Avoid the energy vampires (see page 107) in your life, if possible. If not, try the techniques on page 107 to help you.

- Live and work by your values and beliefs. Remember that your most important relationship is the one you have with yourself.

- Take responsibility for your own feelings, actions and patterns of behaviour.

- Learn to forgive yourself and others. Sometimes letting go of past hurt can release energy.

- Use positive language in everything you do. Make sure your cup is half full, not half empty.

- Don't take yourself too seriously; sometimes we can spend too long in introspective thinking when we should just "go with the flow".

- Consider the energy you receive from food, drink, sunlight and other people, and think of giving it out as well. Make it a gift and visualize handing it out to others who need it.

- Like yourself – think of all the reasons that you are good to be around and reinforce them by standing in front of the mirror and telling yourself why you like yourself.

- Think of yourself as lucky.

BALANCE YOUR LIFE AND WORK

It has been proven that people are more likely to suffer from stress-related sickness when working long hours and not balancing their physical and emotional energies. Stress-related sick leave is at an all-time high in the West. More women with children are now working, with the requirement to fit childcare arrangements within their work practices. People are living longer, meaning an increase in the number of people who are spending time caring for elderly relatives.

Whatever it is that you need from your work and life, just make sure it is in balance. Make changes before you hit crisis point and everything spirals out of control. Consider your work pattern. To what extent is it under your control? Do you follow your plans? Is there room for improvement? Do you take work home? Why? Does it matter?

You may find it helpful to set your alarm clock to go off ten minutes earlier and use that time to prioritize your goals and tasks for the day.

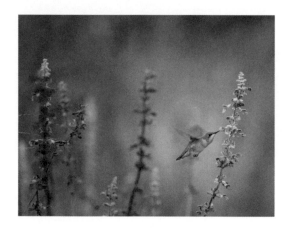

BENEFITS OF A GOOD WORK/LIFE BALANCE

TO YOU	TO YOUR EMPLOYER
The ability to spend time at leisure or other activities	Lower levels of stress-related illness
Time to care for children	Higher morale and motivation
Time to care for elderly relatives	Better staff retention and recruitment
Time to care for disabled people	Increased productivity
A reduction in stress	A wider range of skilled employees
A considerate employer	
Lifestyle choices made by you as an individual	

RELATIONSHIPS WITH COLLEAGUES

Getting along with people at work can be difficult. Even when we fall into an easy friendship with someone, there is still the added complication of having to work with them. If you don't foster good working relations, you will find the situation very energy-sapping. A number of techniques can help you with your relationships with colleagues.

- **Be assertive** – although it is a difficult skill to master, it makes a massive difference to your personal impact (see page 62).

- **Avoid gossip** – office gossip, if it is negative, can lead to bullying. However, do make the most of the office grapevine as usually this proves to be a powerful communication tool.

- **Learn active listening** – this means listening to the words someone is saying without thinking of something else or what you are going to say next. You'll be surprised how many thoughts are going on in your mind at the same time.

- **Negotiate** – but always leave something on the table. All negotiations usually have a winner or a loser, but the ideal solution is where both parties feel that the negotiation is fair.

- **Practise upward management** – you can influence your manager and support their decisions. Don't just wait to be told what to do, but think ahead and manage your own career.

- **Use your powers of influence wisely** – influencing is a skill that can be practised. It is not about coercing, blackmailing or manipulating people, but about how you adapt your behaviour and use excellent communication strategies.

- **Take responsibility** – if you have made a mistake, don't be afraid to stand up and take responsibility for it. It is how you deal and learn from mistakes that is important. If you are in an organization that does not look kindly on people making mistakes, which are part of being human, consider whether this is an organization you are happy within.

- **Use the power of humour** – laughing is a powerful tool, although you must be careful not to use it inappropriately or as a form of bullying.

- **Develop yourself** – understanding yourself and your own behaviours can help you relate to others.

- **Change negative situations** – if you are unhappy with a relationship with one of your colleagues, actively try to change it. Ask for help if necessary.

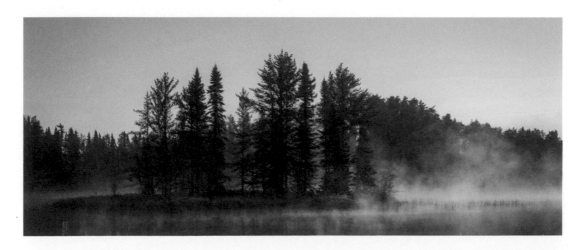

PUT YOUR LIFE IN CONTEXT

The context we live in can have a major effect on our energy levels. Although we choose our friends, we rarely choose our family. However, the family bond is probably one of the strongest ones that we will ever encounter, whether as a child, sibling or parent. Rituals and routines can help manage the hectic side of family life and provide an environment for relationships to flourish.

MANAGING DAILY DEMANDS

Conflicting demands of family, friends or relatives can put heavy demands on our time and energy. Whether it is a routine matter, a sick relative or a needy friend, we can feel pushed and pulled in different directions, resulting in fatigue and stress. Deciding on who to put first when juggling different demands can put a strain on us all. It is important to recognize the reality of what is required versus what you can give. Understanding the toll on your energy and how to stop it happening or finding strategies to replenish energy levels will help you manage your demands.

PERSONAL RELATIONSHIPS

Take time to work on relationships that are important. Often we start relationships with many hopes, yet we end up treating the people we love the most in ways we would not treat strangers. We fail to spend time working on the relationship and making it as good as it can be, and often take others for granted.

The most important element of a successful relationship is communication. Remember the old adage of never going to bed on an argument? Follow the top tips on this page.

KEEP YOUR SENSE OF SELF

It is also possible to lose your sense of self when living in a family context or relationship, and this is incredibly de-energizing. Keeping your roles balanced can be demanding too. For example, when we become parents and find ourselves giving all our energy to young children it is easy to lose sight of ourselves and our needs, causing aspects of our lives, such as sex, to suffer.

TOP TIPS ON RELATIONSHIPS

- Accept people for who they are, not who you think they should be.

- Learn to communicate and listen.

- Be assertive.

- Say sorry when necessary.

- Ask for what you want; don't expect the other person to know.

- Be prepared to compromise.

- Learn to negotiate.

- Avoid criticism; try to focus more on appreciation.

- Respect another's space for being an individual.

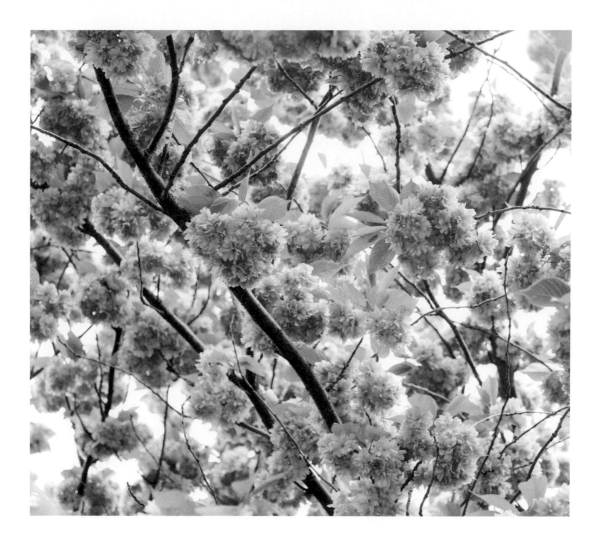

FEMININE AND MASCULINE ENERGIES

Whether you are male or female, you are made up of a mix of feminine and masculine energies. Just as yin and yang shows the seeds of the other within the symbol, so does the feminine hold the masculine within and vice versa. However, social stereotyping has tended to cause masculine words such as "focused", "powerful", "firm", "logical" and "rational" to be considered strong words; and feminine words such as "intuitive", "sensitive", "nurturing", "trusting" and "emotional' to be soft. In the workplace, masculine energy tends to be the energy that is accepted as culturally normal and desirable.

It is important for energies in the world to be in balance, and we need masculine and feminine energy to live in harmony. Neither one is better, but they are different. So how does this relate to you? The key issue is living the energy of who you are in your core being, rather than through learned behaviour or the expectations of society. Remember that you have both energies, but life will feel right when you live your life authentically.

You are more likely to attract and connect to the right partner when you are your true self. You may recognize this as a feeling of "fit" or contentment at an intuitive level, in a similar way to being "in the flow".

LIFE PHASES

You will experience different stages of life, from the very first beginning as a single cell, through birth, childhood, adolescence and the various stages of adulthood. Each of these stages contains its own experiences, and individuals have differing needs at each stage.

IDENTIFY YOUR LIFE STAGE

Interestingly, in energy terms, the process is cyclical in nature, rather than linear. There are peaks and troughs, as in a sine wave, with the length of each peak or trough depending on the environmental aspects at the time.

Which phase are you in currently?

Where would you like to be?

It is fine and natural to travel through the different energy seasons, as long as you don't remain in any one of them for too long. People remaining permanently in the energy winter have little reserves to fall back on and will find a time when they need to refuel.

ENERGY SEASONS

Here are some words that come to mind that are synonymous with the quadrants in the diagram. You may have some of your own as well.

Spring – dependent, starting point, rising energy, fuelling.

Summer – independent, anything is possible, high energy, burning.

Autumn – interdependent, hard graft, falling energy, storing.

Winter – pendent, winding down, low energy, conserving.

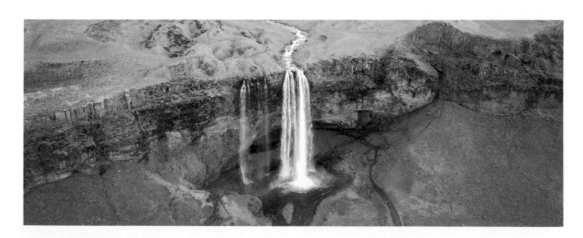

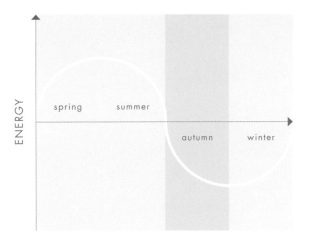

ENERGY

spring   summer

autumn   winter

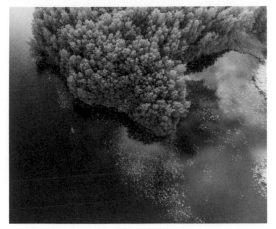

PERSONAL PRIORITIES

Committing to, and living by, a set of values and priorities is completely energizing, as you will find a sense of purpose and feeling of authenticity.

1 Take a piece of paper and write down your values and priorities; try to find ten altogether (a selection is given below but there are many more you could use).

- Achievement
- Balance
- Creativity
- Discipline
- Equality
- Freedom
- Gratitude
- Honesty
- Independence
- Justice
- Knowledge

- Loyalty
- Money
- Openness
- Power
- Quality
- Recognition
- Success
- Trust
- Variety
- Wisdom

2 Out of those ten, choose your top five. These are the five you are going to focus on to make your life more authentic. Put those five in order of importance. This is not an easy task, and will probably take some thought and reflection.

3 The next step is to align your values and priorities with your goals. If you have not already set some, refer back to page 88 for advice on achieving goals. Once you have done this, see whether your values and priorities match your goals.

4 If they do, fantastic! If not, you have two options. You can reconsider your goals, or reconsider your values and priorities. Neither are set in stone; they are flexible and about you choosing what you want from life. If you have a goal that you really want to meet and you need to adopt a new value or priority to reach it, then go ahead and do so. Remember that this is all about your personal power and energy.

SEXUAL IDENTITY

A book on energy would not be complete without discussing sexual energy. We are all sexual beings, whether or not we are in a sexual relationship at the time of reading this book. The overriding issues are being comfortable with yourself, communicating with your partner and exploring your sexual self.

SEXUAL ENERGY

One of the greatest ways of sharing energy between two people is through sex. The energy comes from focusing on your partner, paying attention to their sexual needs and wants, keeping an open mind, communicating and being honest with both your partner and yourself.

Making time for each other and working on your relationship is critical. The difference between having sex as a routine chore rather than as a pleasurable event needs little discussion! Spend time pampering yourself, create the right ambience with candles and aromatherapy, enjoy great food together and make the event one of pure pleasure across all the senses. Be realistic about the energy within you and your partner at that time and either change the environment to harmonize the energies, or choose a different time.

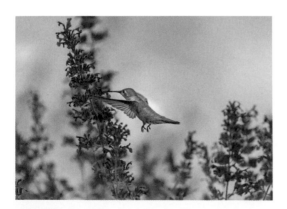

EROTIC MASSAGE

Taking the power of touch one step further, massage can make your partner feel loved, valued and wanted. It has the power to re-energize in an erotic, intimate and giving way.

1 Create a warm and sensual atmosphere with candles and soft music where you won't be disturbed. Start by massaging the shoulders and back, using a base oil with added essential oils to evoke the sense of smell.

2 Roll your partner over and gently massage the front, avoiding the erogenous zones completely. Note what works for your partner and stay focused on the pleasure of the moment.

3 Add scratches and nips if appropriate and increase the tempo, massaging closer and closer to the erogenous zones. Take the massage wherever you and your partner want to.

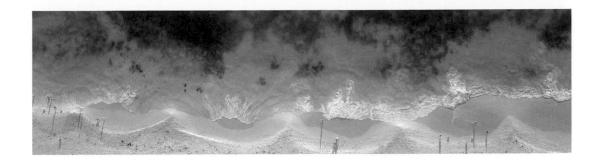

POWER OF TOUCH

Being touched by another human being is one of the most joyful things you can experience in life. Touch varies from gentle to firm, but should always be appropriate. There is nothing like holding hands with someone you love, or hugging, or just curling up on the sofa with some part of your bodies touching.

TANTRIC SEX

Taking energy levels one step further, this is a spiritual way of lovemaking that involves patience and preparation. Rather than focusing solely on orgasm, the emphasis is on the joining of the two individual energy fields in a powerful spiritual and sexual ecstasy, through opening up the chakras (see page 11).

SEXUAL RED FLAGS

Sexual relationships are not always perfect and according to the marriage-guidance organization Relate, these are some common sex problems: sex addiction; being stuck in a rut; difficulty in reaching orgasm; problems with premature ejaculation; partners with different levels of desire; problems getting an erection; painful intercourse and stopping having sex altogether. Don't be afraid to seek external help if any of these apply to you.

TOP TIPS ON EXPRESSING YOUR SEXUAL ENERGY

- Take time for sex.
- Talk about your needs for your sexuality with your partner.
- Flirt.
- Lose your inhibitions and be comfortable in your own skin.
- Dress how you want to dress, not how people want to see you dress.
- Recognize the sexual being within yourself – it is fine to be sexual as a free-willed, consenting adult.
- Realize that our laws reflect our morals and values, which tend to fit in with society norms.
- Understand your partner's sexuality and your own.
- Communicate – not just within the relationship but at a sexual level.
- Listen, watch, discuss – understand what triggers good and bad results.
- Indulge in massage.
- Eat aphrodisiacs – try oysters or chocolate.
- Give your partner a present – not just on a birthday or special occasion.

ENERGY ANGELS AND VAMPIRES

Have you noticed how some people seem to energize the people around them? Energy angels are the people who make you feel amazing and who give you a buzz. On the other hand, sometimes simply talking to someone can make you feel physically drained. These are energy vampires.

ENERGY ANGELS

These people seem to have a natural presence when they walk into a room – almost as if they have an aura of energy. Energy angels tend to speak with positive tones. Their cup is definitely half full, if not completely full! They are already vibrating at a level that is in tune with the rest of the world, even the universe.

The good news is that we can all become an energy angel; it just takes time and practice. Remember: you will attract into your life whatever you think about the most.

BECOME AN ENERGY ANGEL

Visualize yourself as an energy angel. Imagine you are bathed in a white light. See the white light carrying the energy leave your body and freely share it with anyone around you. As you give out the energy, imagine you are tapped into the complete energy of the universe. Focus on that for a while and, as it becomes easier, you will be surprised at the results.

Visualization works because the mind doesn't know the difference between waking reality, dreams or consciously directed visualization. The mind understands all of these experiences as if it were a waking experience. We use our conscious selves to determine the difference between

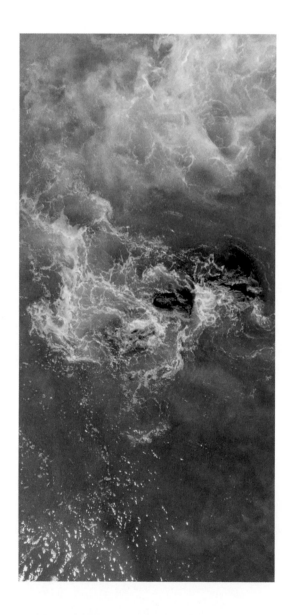

normal waking reality and the dream world, but to our subconscious, they are the same.

Once you have conquered the imagination, you will find that giving energy to others becomes second nature. Giving away energy will not deplete you as there is an unlimited amount. Instead, you will find you start to attract a different type of person. You will discover more energy in the people you mix with and recognize other energy angels. Imagine yourself as resonating at a different vibrational level, attracting others at similar vibrations.

ENERGY VAMPIRES

Spend a few moments thinking about people you interact with and see if you can identify anyone who drains your energy. We all have moments in life where we are in need of others and perhaps become energy vampires ourselves.

How can you step out of this? Start with the basic technique below – it is all about maintaining control of your own energy and choosing your behaviour rather than being sucked into someone else's need.

The advanced conquering technique gives you the tools you need to help give energy to the individual concerned.

BEAT THE VAMPIRE!

The basic technique. This may take a bit of practice, but it is worth persevering with.

- You have just realized that the person you are with is draining your energy. Stop for a moment and look inside yourself. Where is the feeling – in the pit of your stomach, chest or head? Is it stationary or moving somewhere else?

- Take that feeling and imagine it fizzling away. Use your mind until it has completely disappeared. Imagine a bright, white light filling the space you have just made. Think of the light as never-ending and start to see it freely passing from you to the other person.

- Keep your body energized. Stand or sit up tall, keep your chin up and your shoulders relaxed. Breathe deeply and calmly.

- If you find yourself becoming angry, upset or out of control, distance yourself from your emotions. Imagine that this is happening to someone else and you are watching from afar.

CONQUER THE VAMPIRE!

The advanced technique. Once you have practised and mastered the basic technique, you can try this one.

- Match the other person's body language, their tone and speed of voice, mirror their movements and try to breathe at the same rate they do. This creates a subconscious empathy with the other person.

- After a while, start to change the way you talk, move and breathe. If speech was fast, slow it down and vice versa. Change your posture to an energized one – do this at a rate that brings the other person with you and starts to lift them too.

- Focus your language on positives. Inject some humour, if appropriate, to the situation – which will release feel-good endorphins.

- All the time, imagine that a bright, white light is passing into you, through you and freely into the other person (see "Become an energy angel" on the opposite page).

SPIRITUAL ENERGY TECHNIQUES

Spirituality means different things to different people. It may be something that is important to you or you may not see yourself as a spiritual person. Spirituality is about understanding one's self and that there is more that connects us than the material world around us. People may see it as another dimension. My understanding of spirituality is that it encompasses having clearly defined values, maintaining compassion and empathy for oneself and others, and feeling a sense of purpose, that there is more to life. You will have your own understanding of spirituality.

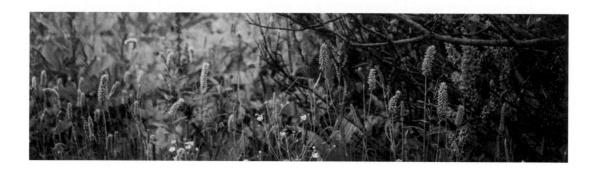

FINDING SPIRITUALITY

Walk into a place of beauty or watch an electric thunderstorm – these can cause you to be filled with an overwhelming feeling of spirituality. Places of worship often have a sense of spirituality; this may be because they are places of worship, or because their locations were chosen for their innate sense of spirituality. "Ley lines", which also inspire feelings of spirituality, are said to be alignments of Earth energy that connect various sacred sites.

There are many religions and faiths, which all have their own spiritual teachings. This is not a book about religion, but it is essential to recognize its place and importance, in accordance with your own beliefs.

GROWTH AND DEVELOPMENT

Life has many challenges and it is the way you deal with them that provides the opportunity for personal growth. We make a myriad of decisions every day. Some decisions feel impossible, and others seem irrelevant, but they all have consequences. We often don't know what the consequences will be, and they may be significant or unimportant, immediate or long term, stand-alone or bound up with many other decisions.

Many people assist us through life; our parents, teachers, mentors and coaches, who influence us in subtle ways. There is a saying that "when the pupil is ready, the teacher appears". However, you need to grasp those opportunities for growth when they arrive. Remember, we sometimes learn most from the situations that are most challenging and difficult.

Where does that leave us? If part of our purpose in life is to grow, there are two critical areas for development: overcoming negative habit patterns and building self-esteem.

OVERCOME NEGATIVE HABIT PATTERNS

As discussed in other sections of this book, the first step is awareness. Write down any negative habit patterns you can think of (behaviour such as manipulation, procrastination, being over-sensitive, loudness). Examine what motivates you to use each of these habits and analyse the consequences of your behaviour in this respect.

Now you are aware, all you need to do is change things. Next time you find you are adopting a negative habit pattern, stop, walk away or try a different type of behaviour. It will take a while to change, but it is possible. You are already halfway there just recognizing your negative habits.

Some people find writing down what has happened, their response and the outcome helpful. Look back over six or seven areas and plan how to manage events differently. Others learn from talking through their experiences with friends and asking for advice or taking time for self-reflection.

If your negative behaviour patterns are deep-rooted, it may be that you need to get help with recognizing and overcoming these patterns in order to change them to a positive.

BUILD YOUR SELF-ESTEEM

Self-esteem is about how you value yourself. Low self-esteem can be built up through being treated badly by others or by thinking badly of yourself. The impact of low self-esteem should not be taken lightly, as it can affect your happiness, health and success.

- Set yourself a goal right now, and make that goal one of looking after you! Put yourself as the number one, because it is only by looking after your own needs and wants that you can in turn give energy to others.

- Use the meditation, breathing and relaxation techniques in this book. Lie in a bath with candles. If the voice in your head starts to tell you negative things, switch it off. Write a list of everything that is good about you and read it to yourself every morning.

- Remember that you are an amazing person and the first person that needs to know that is you.

- Surround yourself with people who help you to feel good about yourself.

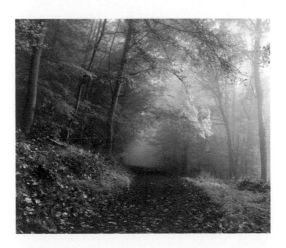

MIND, BODY AND SPIRIT

Seeing yourself as a holistic whole, with your mind, body and spirit in balance, gives you a sense of authenticity about who you are. You will have a sense of well-being, peace and a connection with yourself as an individual and as part of a greater whole.

A BALANCING ACT

However, we frequently act out of balance in our everyday lives, perhaps focusing on our work and ignoring our physical needs. The sections on intellectual energy and physical energy techniques cover tips for improving these. Yet, even if we spend a lot of time balancing our mind and body, the spirit can often be left behind. How balanced are you?

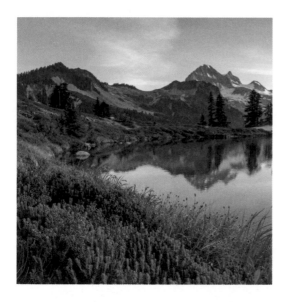

ARE YOU IN BALANCE?

1 Write notes under each of these headings to explore how you run your life (some ideas are suggested):
Mind Analyzing, organizing, generating ideas
Body Exercise, movement, getting results I can see
Spirit Intuitive, inspired, aware of my purpose

2 Then write down what it is you avoid in these three areas.

3 Are the three aspects balanced? If they are, congratulations, but you probably were aware of this already. If not, think about how you could bring them closer together. One of the most powerful ways to put yourself in balance is by meditating. You will find some meditations on pages 116–117.

Next time you are feeling negative emotions – for example, when you are nervous about an interview – try the following technique.

1 Take a deep breath and imagine that breath is puffing you up like a balloon. Feel yourself getting taller and your body expanding into the space around you. Focus on that feeling with each breath you take.

2 Feel the emotion inside you and allow it to spread around your veins, changing the feeling to one of power and energy.

3 Visualize yourself as taller, stronger and in complete control of the emotion.

4 Walk taller and with body language that believes this is true.

5 Now you have connected your mind and body, feel the freedom of your spirit.

REGAIN YOUR BALANCE

When you are going to a busy city, how do you feel? Is your energy being sapped? It is easier to balance yourself in a quiet room or a quiet forest when the sounds are natural than in a city filled with discordant traffic sounds where you are being bombarded with mixed energies from different sources.

Stop for a moment and remember a time when you felt sad or upset about something. Recapture that emotion and see how you are sitting or standing. Think of your body language. Now think of another time, but one where you felt happy and on top of the world. What is your body language like now? Compare the difference between the two, and consider if your emotions can affect your physical demeanour. Imagine how changing your physical bearing can alter your emotions.

FLOWER ESSENCES

These provide a natural way to help you overcome emotional issues. The idea is that a healthy mind leads to a healthy body, so it connects the mind, body and spirit. Bach Original Flower Remedies have been used for 70 years and include 38 different remedies for problems in seven groups: fear; loneliness; uncertainty; lack of interest; despondency and despair; too much concern for others; oversensitivity. There is also a remedy called "Rescue Remedy" designed to calm you.

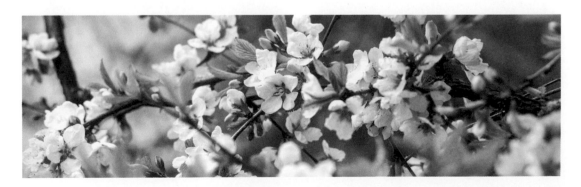

PATHS TO SPIRITUAL FULFILMENT

Have you ever thought about a certain person – then a moment later the phone rings and they are on the other end? Have you met someone who, whatever is happening around them, seems to have an overall understanding, just by sensing? Have you ever had a gut feeling about something? This is intuition. Learning to understand and develop it enhances your spiritual energy.

FIND YOUR INTUITION

Stop for a moment and think about a time where you had an unconscious understanding of an event or a person. Did you listen to that feeling? Did you act on it or let it influence your decision-making?

Write down a question and start writing your answer – don't stop and think about it, but allow your mind to flow and write down everything that you think. Don't re-read what you have written, but follow on with another question and another question until you have nothing else to write. (If you struggle with this, refer to the creativity technique on pages 86–87.) True intuition is immediate and unforced.

TOP TIPS ON DEVELOPING YOUR INTUITION

• Keep an intuition diary – scribble down thoughts as they come to you and see what happens.

• Listen to yourself.

• Watch and listen to others.

• Meditate.

INCREASE YOUR EMPATHY

What is empathy? The dictionary defines it as "a feeling of concern and understanding for another's situation or feelings". Increase your empathy by taking time out to focus on other people and listen to them. Here are some guidelines for increasing your empathy:

• Put yourself in the other person's shoes – use your own memories to connect and link.

• Imagine how you would feel, but don't impose your feelings.

• Ask questions so that you have a greater understanding.

• Practise active listening but don't give solutions; instead focus on their feelings.

• Be non-judgemental.

• Find a good empathetic role model and model your behaviour on theirs.

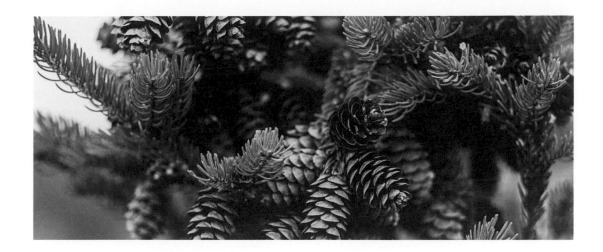

BUILD YOUR COMPASSION

Compassion is similar to empathy, but takes it one step further. It links to suffering and the desire to reduce another's suffering. It is about being connected with other living beings and unconditional love. The more we care for others, the more inner peace we gain and the greater our ability to be compassionate. However, be aware that true compassion is difficult to come by as we are naturally interested in our own needs and it is easy to mix compassion with neediness.

Start to build your compassionate nature, by replacing feelings of anger and hate with love, reason and patience. Have the intention to become more truly compassionate and you will find your compassion increasing. Treat everyone you come across with compassion; have it at the forefront of your mind.

TAKE RESPONSIBILITY

In several religions, the concept of "karma" says that all your deeds, good and bad, will have consequences in your life. It includes intentional actions, whether they are mental, verbal or physical. It is the law of cause and effect, so take responsibility for your own thoughts and actions.

CONSIDER YOURSELF LUCKY

Adopt an attitude of feeling lucky. Studies have shown that, while people are generally no more lucky or unlucky than someone else, individuals who think they are more lucky take more risks and grasp more opportunities in life.

BE WISE

Wisdom comes from experience rather than being something we are born with. It is in the mind and is made up of self-knowledge, judgement and insight. The more you experience life and become self-aware, the wiser you will become.

LIVE IN THE MOMENT

It is easy to spend time focusing on what has been or dreaming about what is going to be. Often past memories that we focus on are negative ones. Try spending time living in the moment and focus on what you are doing now.

COMPLEMENTARY ENERGIZERS

The most holistic energizer has already been mentioned in this book – a combination of adequate sleep, good nutrition and sensible exercise. However, assuming that this is something you are already achieving, there are also complementary energizers that work well to maintain balance.

COLOUR THERAPY

Colour affects our energy, and colour therapy is a way of using the colours to improve our overall well-being. The chakras (see page 11) all have a colour associated with them. You can carry out colour therapy on yourself by meditating on the colour that you feel you need or feel most drawn to, using the following chart. Surround yourself with colours, remembering that balance is key.

SOUND THERAPY

In a similar way to colour therapy, sound therapy is about unblocking the chakras to improve our energy levels. This can be using modern instruments or more unusual means such as Tibetan singing bowls, gongs and chanting voices.

BE STILL

Our minds are active all the time; even while we sleep, the brain produces dreams. Finding time to be still and do nothing for a moment is incredibly energizing. However, it is not easy for most of us, so try the following technique to help you. Use the breath to calm the mind – this will both give you peace and improve your self-discipline and willpower. It will take practice and you will discover how busy your mind can be – it deserves a rest too.

1 Sit in a comfortable chair in a room or place where you will not be disturbed and close your eyes.

2 Gently inhale and exhale through your nose, focusing on the breath and being aware of the sensation as it travels through your nose, down into your lungs and then back out through your nose.

3 Keep focusing on your breath and, if thoughts come into your mind, let them go.

4 If thoughts keep coming, start to count each breath, silently. See how far you can count without any other thoughts encroaching. Sit, calmly breathing, for a minimum of 3 minutes.

COLOUR	CHAKRA	ASSOCIATED WITH
Red	Root	Vitality, courage, self-confidence, danger, strength, power, passion, desire, love.
Orange	Sacral	Happiness, confidence, resourcefulness, enthusiasm, fascination, happiness, creativity, determination, attraction, success, encouragement, stimulation.
Yellow	Solar plexus	Wisdom, clarity, self-esteem, joy, happiness, intellect.
Green	Heart	Balance, love, self-control, growth, harmony, freshness, safety, fertility.
Blue	Throat	Knowledge, health, decisiveness, depth, stability, trust, loyalty, wisdom, confidence, intelligence, faith, truth.
Indigo	Third eye	Intuition, mysticism, nobility, luxury, ambition, wealth, mystery.
Violet	Crown	Beauty, creativity, inspiration.

HERBAL REMEDIES

The following remedies can be used to alleviate the effects of various physical and mental problems and facilitate the flow of energy. They are not a substitute for seeking medical advice if you are unwell.

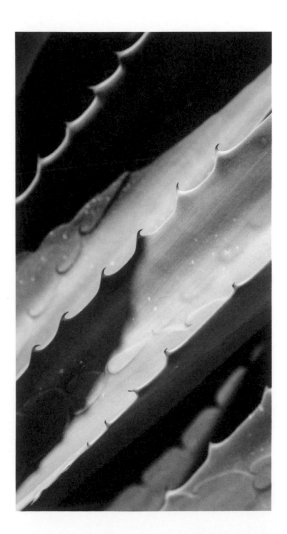

- Aloe vera – good for minor burns

- Chamomile – aids digestion

- Cranberry – good for urinary-tract infections

- Echinacea – boosts the immune system

- Feverfew – good for migraines

- Flaxseed – good for hot flushes and osteoporosis

- Garlic – acts as an antibiotic

- Ginger – good for sickness

- Ginkgo – improves circulation to the brain

- Lavender – good for anxiety

- Peppermint – to settle the stomach

- St John's wort – good for depression and anxiety

- Tea tree oil – acts as an antiseptic

MEDITATION

Meditation has been used as a tool to balance the mind, body and spirit for thousands of years. It is about focusing or stilling your mind, whether by being still, listening to guided meditation or chanting mantras. It has been used both within religions and for spiritual growth and is recognized by modern-day doctors as a powerful relaxation technique and as a preventative form of therapy.

BENEFITS OF MEDITATING

It is reported that brain scans of Buddhist meditation masters have recorded jumps of over 700 per cent in neural activity in the areas of the brain related to happiness compared to just over 10 per cent for people new to meditation. Meditation has many benefits, including promoting relaxation, increasing self-awareness and self-knowledge, improving self-discipline and encouraging serenity.

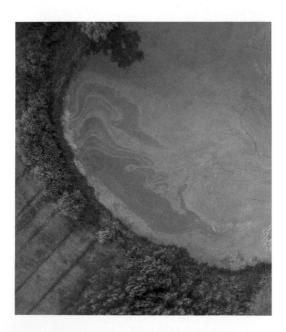

STARTING TO MEDITATE

If you have not meditated before, try the following technique.

1   Find a quiet, calm place to sit down, either on a chair or on the floor. Close your eyes and relax your body. Breathe slowly and count each breath.

2   When thoughts come into your mind, let them pass by, continuing to focus on your breath.

3   Keep counting until you reach 100 (but don't worry if you lose count; the important issue is to keep your focus, so just start again at 1).

4   After a few minutes, stop counting and slowly start to focus on the environment around you.

5   Slowly open your eyes and give yourself a moment to reorientate yourself before standing up.

Don't expect to be able to still your mind immediately; it takes practice. However, you will feel the benefit in your energy levels straight away.

USING MUSIC

When you are happy with your meditation, try introducing appropriate meditative music to your practice. There is a great deal of suitable music available to purchase or download.

CHANTING

Meditation does not always mean silent reflection. Typically, Buddhists chant mantras to unite the breath, mind and voice. This calms the body by focusing on one thing only. Whether you consider that the choice of mantra you chant is important will depend on your personal beliefs, but whatever you choose those words will receive your focus for as long as you are chanting. You could try chanting, "Namu Myoho Renge Kyo" – to obey, to adore and to devote to the universal laws; "Om" – a sacred exclamation; or "Om Namah Shivaya" – I bow to Shiva (Shiva is the supreme reality, the inner Self).

INTERMEDIATE MEDITATION

As you become more practised at your meditative routines, you will be able to focus on balancing your energies. Relax your body and sit in a comfortable, straight, steady posture. Don't let yourself be disturbed, but maintain a clear focus within. As the thoughts come and you let go, consider how useful they are and allow your conscious mind to note those thoughts that are of benefit to you right now.

ADVANCED MEDITATION

In advanced meditation, you move beyond the realm of focusing on breath or mantras and feel your part within what is known as the "universal energy". You may have no need for mantras but will be able to take yourself to a higher plane without thought. It is stillness, serenity, self-realization.

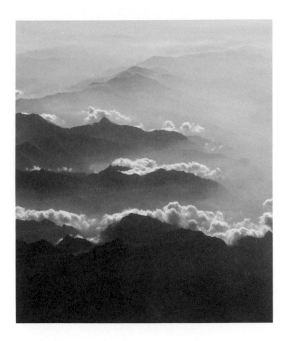

WALKING MEDITATION

If you find it difficult to keep still, or would like to try a different type of meditation, try this walking meditation.

1 As you take a step forward, breathe in. As you take the next step, breathe out.

2 Continue to step and breathe at a slow, measured pace, counting each step as you take it.

3 When thoughts come into your mind, let them pass by, continuing to focus on your breath and your step.

4 Keep your focus soft so that, while you can see where you are going, you are not actively looking at anything.

5 Keep the breath and step synchronized and your mind quiet for at least 5 minutes.

VISUALIZATION TECHNIQUES

Visualization is about using your mind to see something you want, with the aim of using the visualization to make you feel better, give you more energy or to help you reach your goals. Some creative visualization exercises have already been described (see pages 94–95) for developing a morning ritual and making a dream board.

HOW TO VISUALIZE

It is important to learn to relax (use the relaxation technique on page 67 to help). Start to visualize by using your brain to imagine a picture of what it is that you want. This does not necessarily mean you can see something like a picture on a television.

Start with something simple – try these two quick exercises to practise before you start in earnest. Read each of the following through first, then close your eyes and describe your visualization out loud:

Your front door – what colour is it, where is the door handle, how do you approach it?

Your bedroom – where is the bed, what colour are the walls, what furniture is in there?

How does visualization work for you? Did you see a picture or was it more of a sense of knowing? Once you are confident with your ability to visualize (whether you can see or not), move on to this next exercise:

- Think of something you want, close your eyes and picture it how you would like it to be.

- Make the picture as real and colourful as possible.

- Fill it with emotion, and make it as big and bright as possible.

- Make it a moving picture, if possible.

- Keep seeing or playing your picture or movie at frequent intervals during the day.

- Have complete belief that this is making its way to you. What do you have to lose?

Your ability will improve with practice. Remember what the law of attraction states – you attract that which you focus on. So, bring to mind the things that you want out of life and think about them often.

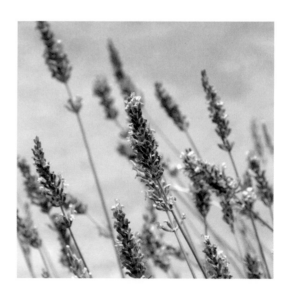

VISUALIZE FOR WELL-BEING

1 Start by using the simple meditation exercise on page 116 to relax yourself.

2 Imagine a sense of peace and calm start to fall upon your body with each breath.

3 See it as a cleansing light that unblocks energy in all seven of your chakras (see page 11), one by one.

4 Think of the light as white, and then break down the light and visualize the seven distinct colours of the rainbow, one by one, passing around your body healing, energizing and making you feel fantastic.

5 After some time, let the colours merge back into a white light and feel it gently leave you full of energy and well-being.

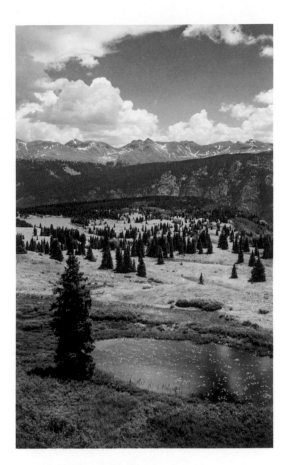

VISUALIZE FOR SUCCESS

1 Focus on whatever it is that you want to be successful in or with (this works well with the goal-setting technique on page 88).

2 Close your eyes and imagine yourself as having that success right now.

3 Picture it exactly as you would if you could make wishes come true.

4 Imagine how successful you feel – picture the prize or goal as it comes towards you.

5 Enjoy the moment and come back to it time and time again.

VISUALIZE FOR RELAXATION

1 See yourself as being relaxed. Imagine you are in a spa retreat or a place of great beauty.

2 Close your eyes and allow the sensation of peace to fall over you.

3 Hear the sound of the ocean or the sound of birds calling to each other from the trees.

4 Allow yourself to fall deeper into the relaxing sensations as your body becomes heavier.

5 Feel the benefit to your body, mind and spirit.

ENERGY, HERE I COME!

This book will only be as good as the work you put into it. Despite how motivated you may feel, you should be aware that often, when starting out on a voyage of self-development, there will be things that get in the way and people who will try to stop you. You may even inhibit yourself. Don't worry about this. Acknowledge that it is the case, and accept it. It is partly how you deal with these setbacks that really tests you. Use the following pages to help you plan and take your first steps, to make new habits and to create a sustainable, energized future.

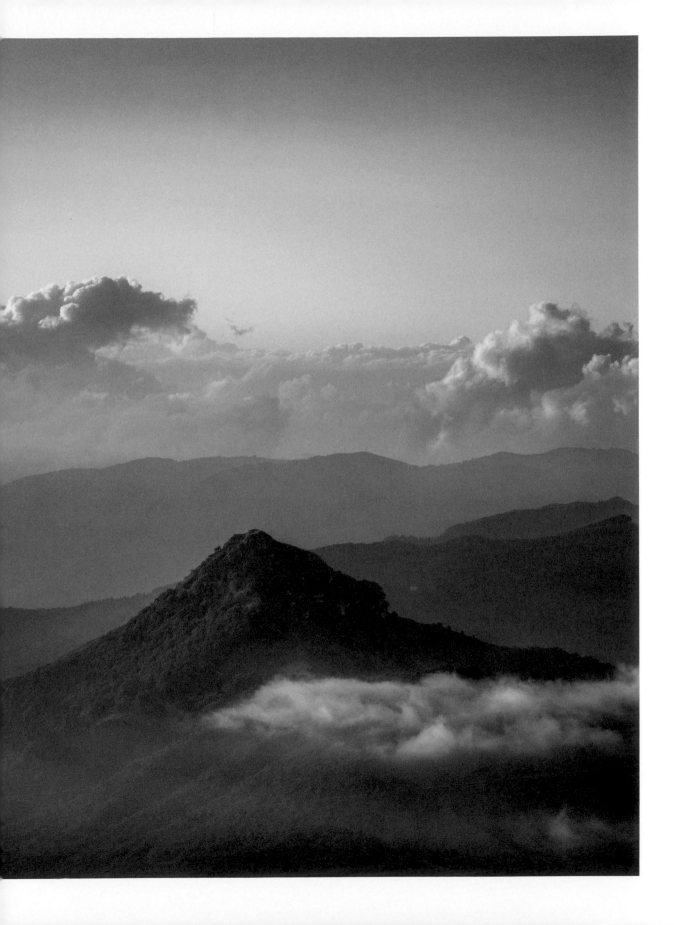

TAKING THE FIRST STEP

Going on a journey can seem a long and challenging task, however exciting and thrilling it may be. However, every journey has to start with a single step and taking one step is easy. Fill in the planning tool below to help you take your first step.

Make sure you feel balanced and energized before you start. Be honest with yourself and remember, the more you put into the exercise, the more you will gain from it. Use the knowledge you have gained from reading through the book to help you.

PLAN YOUR JOURNEY

What are my current strengths?

What have I achieved so far?

What do I need or want to develop?

What or who might help me?

What or who might stop me?
What can I do to prevent this?

What are my priorities?

Where and when am I going to start?

How will I judge my success?

I KNOW WHAT I MEAN BY ENERGY

○ I have answered the questionnaire and drawn my overall energy profile

○ I have considered my energy balance

My primary focus is on:

○ Physical energy

○ Emotional energy

○ Intellectual energy

○ Creative energy

○ Personal energy

○ Spiritual energy

My secondary focus is on:

○ Physical energy

○ Emotional energy

○ Intellectual energy

○ Creative energy

○ Personal energy

○ Spiritual energy

○ I have completed the planning tool

○ I have set clear objectives and goals

○ I have set myself a time plan

○ I have set rewards on my path

○ I have built a support network to help me

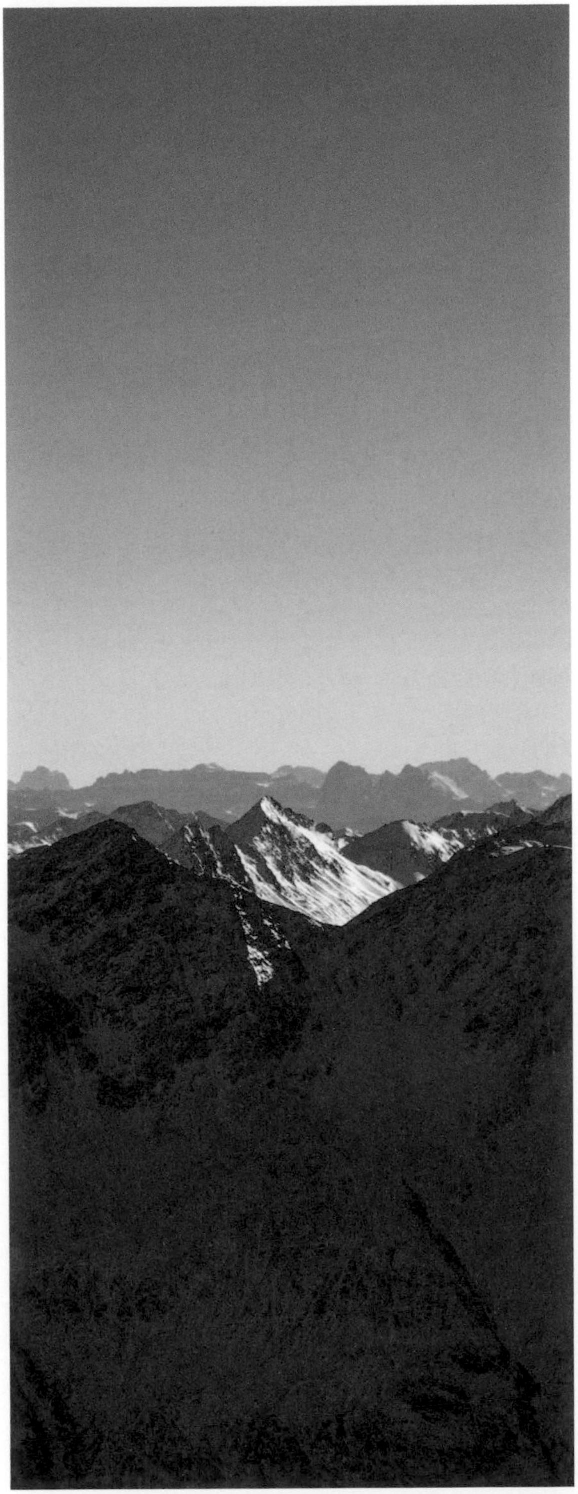

MAINTAIN YOUR ENERGY

This is a book about owning and managing your energy and, by now, assuming that you have incorporated some of the knowledge you have gained and practised some of the techniques, you should have seen some major improvements in your energy levels. The next step is to make sure that this is for life, by incorporating the following.

STOP THE LEAKS

We all need to discharge waste from our bodies, and it is just as important to remove any negative energies from our mind, body and spirit. Removing this unwanted waste is a critical part of managing our energy, but we also need to make sure we don't lose all the positive stuff we have been working on.

When situations, people or the environment start to affect your energy in an attempt to drain it away, make a conscious effort to stop the leaks. Distance yourself and imagine yourself as a conduit that only allows negative energy to escape; hold a swirling, white light of energy around you.

RECHARGE FOR FREE

Once you have stopped any leaks, consider how you can give your energy out for free. Take your swirling, white image of energy and imagine that it is continuously replenished. This can be from the air via the top of your head or through the ground via your feet. Whatever your image is, imagine the energy flooding in as if you are plugged into the energy source like a rechargeable battery. Once you have unlimited energy coming in, just think of the potential energy you can give out.

MAKE IT A HABIT

Habits are unconscious behaviour patterns learned through repetitive and frequent actions. Therefore, to make our good energy techniques into habits, we need to repeat them frequently, giving ourselves lots of positive reinforcement on the way. Think, for example, of how you can now start a car and drive without thinking about it, yet remember how much effort you had to put in when you began to learn to drive. Set yourself a goal to make maintaining high, positive energy levels key to your life, and reward yourself along the way.

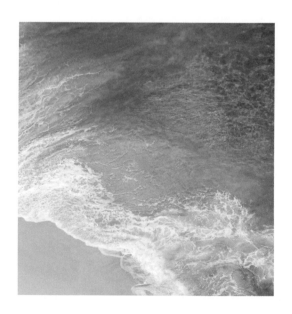

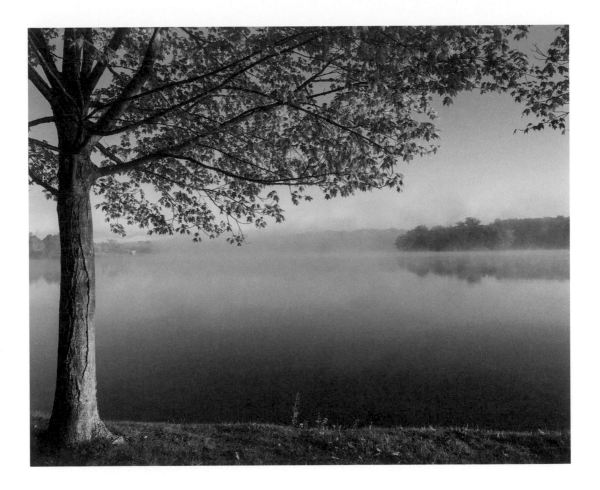

RENEWABLE AND SUSTAINABLE ENERGY

You can generate goodwill by giving energy out. It does not have to be an exchange, but in its own way you are banking energy and storing it for the future. Think of the way that composting waste allows important nutrients to go back into the ground to be used for the next growth cycle. Consider your giving and sharing of energy in a similar way; it is all part of a renewable and sustainable future.

ENERGY MANAGEMENT

Recognizing the massive demands of 21st-century living and the exhaustion that comes with it, by acting on the advice in this book, you should now be living a different, energized life. That does not mean that it is by any means perfect, but you are much further along your road to personal fulfilment.

Would you rather receive or give energy? Are you no longer dependent on others for energy fixes? We get energy all the time from our food, drink and the environment. Think also about how much energy you are giving out to others.

There is a buzz about using things in an appropriate way. The skill of recycling, living harmoniously with the universe and using the Earth's energy rather than fighting against it is an amazing gift.

Enjoy the energy it brings.

INDEX

acupuncture 10
aerobic exercise 54
ageing 19
alcohol 51, 64
anchoring 15
angels, energy 106–7
anger 61, 63
appropriate energy 16
aromatherapy 79
assertiveness 62, 99
avoidance 62
Ayurvedic medicine 10–11

Bach Original Flower
  Remedies 111
balance 110–11
behaviour habits 14, 64–5,
  109, 124–5
biorhythms 18
blockages 92–3
blood-sugar levels 76
"blues" 67–8
body mass index (BMI) 48
brain, intellectual energy
  34–5, 72–83
brainstorming 44, 87
breakfast 50
breathing 56–7

caffeine 50
calories 48, 49
carbohydrates 52–3
chakras 11, 115
chanting 117
chi 11
childbirth 19
children 45
clutter 78
colour therapy 114–15
compassion 113
complementary energizers
  114–15
constraints 45

context, putting your life in
  100–1
creative energy 36–7, 84–95

dehydration 51
depression 18, 68
detoxing 51
diet 48–9, 50–3, 76–7
dream board 95
drinks
  alcohol 51, 64
  energy drinks 53
  smoothies 53
  water 51

emotional energy 32–3,
  60–71
emotional freedom therapy
  (EFT) 62
empathy 112
endorphins 64
energy angels 106–7
energy deficit 75
energy equation 14, 48
energy profiles 23–45
energy vampires 107
energy zone 11
erotic massage 104
essential fatty acids 76
exercise 16, 54–5, 64
expectations 16–17
experiencing energy 15

fats, in diet 51
fear 61, 92
feel-good factors 64–5
feminine energies 101
flexibility training 54
flow/zone 11
flower essences 111
food 48–9, 50–3, 76–7

glycaemic index (GI) 52–3

goals 88–9

habits 14, 64, 109, 124–5
hangovers 51
hate 61
head massage 11
headstand 81
herbal remedies 115
high-energy foods 51
hunger 50

illness 45
Indian head massage 11
influence, sphere of 17
insomnia 45
intellectual energy 34–5,
  72–83
intelligence 73
intuition 112

learning styles 82–3
leisure 74–5
lemon oil 79
life phases 19, 102–3
life/work balance 98–9
living in the moment 113
love 61
luck 113

magnesium 76
maintaining energy 124–5
masculine energies 101
massage 12
  endorphins 64
  erotic massage 104
  Indian head massage 11
meditation 116–17
Mediterranean diet 77
memory 73, 83
menopause 19
mental exercises 82–3
meridians 10, 11, 12, 62
minerals 76

mood swings 68–9
morning ritual 94
motivation 55
muscles 54, 57–9
music 117

negative energies 124
negative habits 109

obesity 45
omega-3 fatty acids 76
omega-6 fatty acids 76
oxygen 79

personal energy 38–9,
96–107
personal fulfilment 17
physical energy 30–1, 48–59
physical well-being 20–1, 49,
119
plants 79
pollution 79
portion sizes 50
positive energy 62–3
positive thinking 12, 96–7
posture 57, 78
pregnancy 19
priorities, personal 103
pseudo-energy 14

Qigong 12

the Rabbit 80
recharging batteries 14, 124
red flags 20–1, 105
reflection and awareness

technique 74
Reiki 12
relationships
with colleagues 99
personal 100
sexual energy 104
relaxation 66–7, 119
renewable energy 125
responsibility, taking 113
rest 66–7

salt 51
saturated fats 51
science 12
seasonal affective disorder
(SAD) 18
seasons, energy 102–3
self, sense of 100
self-esteem 109
serotonin 65
sexual energy 104
shiatsu 12
shift patterns, work 45
sleep 45, 66–7
smoothies 53
snacks 51
sound therapy 114
sphere of influence 17
spiritual energy 40–1, 108–19
stillness 114
strength training 54
stress 20, 70–1, 98
stretching 57–9
success, visualization exercise 119
sugar 50
sustainable energy 125

synchronicity 12

Tai Chi 13
tantric sex 105
time/energy ratio 75
time management 90–1
time zones, travel and 45
touch 105
travel 45

universal energy 13

vampires, energy 107
visualization 94–5, 118–19
vitamins 76

walking meditation 117
warning signals 20–1, 105
water, drinking 51
weight gain 45
weight loss 48
well-being 20–1, 49, 119
wisdom 113
work 74–5
constraints 45
environment 78
relationships with
colleagues 99
work/life balance 75, 98–9
writer's block 92

yin and yang 13, 101
yoga 69, 93

zinc 76

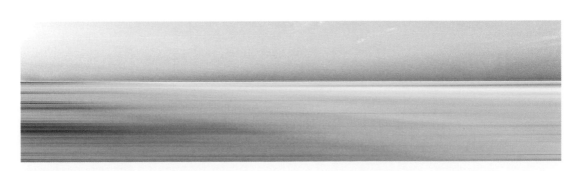

ACKNOWLEDGEMENTS

AUTHOR ACKNOWLEDGEMENTS

I would like to thank my family and friends, whose unconditional love fills me with energy and joy every day and who are always there on the other end of the telephone through the ups and downs that life brings. I especially thank two incredibly amazing women – Chris and Vicky Salter – who have spent late nights listening to my ideas as well as sharing their own. Without them this book would be less than it is. I also thank Dan McCarthy who firmly set me on my path.

PICTURE CREDITS

Dreamstime.com Milosz Aniol 33. **freeimages. com** Kimberly Vohsen 11. **Octopus Publishing Group** Mike Good 56 right, 57, 58, 69, 80, 93. **Unsplash** Aaron Burden 125; Adrien Olichon 43; Amber Teasley 67; Amy Humphries 97; Anthony Cantin 127; Ben Maguire 88; Naomi Hutchinson 41; Atik Sulianami 9; Banter Snaps 90; Benny Jackson 15; Bernard Hermant 25; Brady Bellini 117; Sergey Pesterev 50; Mike Castro Demaria 45; Candre Mandawe 102; Dan Gold 49; Daria Tumanova 6; Dawid Zawila 12; Deanna Alys 63; Diana Macesanu 68; Willian Justen de Vasconcellos 37; Donald Giannatti 119; Aditya Ali 72; Fernando Reyes 128; Janine Joles 118; Frank Mckenna 56 left; Greta Farnedi 108; Guillaume Briard 13; Guy Bowden 10; Hanson Lu 106; John Hernandez 82; Humphrey Muleba 103; Ian Dooley 65; Arkadiusz Zet 60; Jamie Davies 4-5; Jeremy Bishop 73; Reinis Birznieks 124; Jonas Verstuyft 84; Juan Davila 99; Kari Shea 91; Lachlan Gowen 77; Elena Prokofyeva 86; lee 47; Jingda Chen 110; Lorenzo Spoleti 121; Marion Michele 23, 31; Kai Oberhauser 123; Mathew Smith 105; Meric Dagli 78; Miguel Bruna 115; Nathan Dumlao 39; Osman Rana 113; Pablo Garcia Saldana 53; Patrick Brinksma 116; Paul Gilmore 61; Quino Al 19; Ray Hennessy 98; Rodion Kutsaev 89; Andrea Reiman 104; Rupert Britton 95; Scott Webb 92; Sebastian Unrau 109; Sergee Bee 29; Gabriel Garcia Marengo 101; Shifaaz Shamoon 87; Sole D Alessandro 94; Mathyas Kurmann 96; Thomas Rey 79; Tim Gouw 111; Tomoko Uji 20; Trevor Cole 75; Will Swann 35.

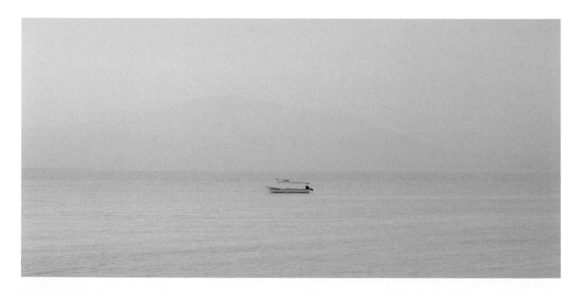